To Kathleen and Richard,
for many happy
hours of reading.
    Love,
    Barbara and Margaret

July 15, 1994

A SENSE OF HUMAN

A SENSE OF HUMAN

Observations about life
by News-Sentinel columnist
Ina Hughs

▓ The Knoxville News-Sentinel

Cover design by Martin Gehring
Back cover photograph by J. Miles Cary

CONTENTS

IV. FAMILY AND OTHER FRUSTRATIONS

V. WONDERS OF HEAVEN AND EARTH

VI. A BUFFET OF HOLIDAYS

VII. CRAZY PEOPLE AND OTHER SOUTHERN PHENOMENA

VIII. ADVENTURES ELSEWHERE

IX. . . . FROM THE BACK OF THE CLOSET

FOREWORD

This book represents a collection of writings by Ina Hughs, general interest columnist for The Knoxville News-Sentinel.

Since she joined The News-Sentinel in 1989, Ina has infuriated many readers, but probably not as many as she has entertained and satisfied. Our letter writers have called her a "beacon of light" and a "flaming heathen-left liberal." Even a "femi-nazi."

I don't know that I would call her any of those things. I *do* call her the only person in our newsroom whose books and belongings take up *two* cubicles instead of one. I *don't* call her the best speller we have on staff. But I *do* think she deserves extra points for building me a model fire truck to add to my collection.

In the spring of 1993, when she won her second Golden Press Card award for columns, contest judges said her entry demonstrated "good, crisp writing . . . imaginative with lively use of images and concrete detail. The columns have a nice, spirited flow . . ."

Regardless of how you tag her or her work, Ina is someone special. She is in demand to speak at club meetings and civic events. She had been with The News-Sentinel only about a year when we assigned her to doing three columns a week for Page Two. She also writes human interest features and a collection of briefs called Sunday Sampler for the Sunday Perspective section. For a year or more, she did a column of trivia and such for our Living section, which we called For Starters.

"A Sense of Human" is a scrapbook of Ina's best work from all the above sources. A few of the pieces which appear in the book originally were published, in one form or another, in The Charlotte Observer or The Charleston Post and Courier. Ina had worked for both of those newspapers before joining the staff of The News-Sentinel.

We enjoy Ina's columns and know that many of our readers share her compassion, humor and her "Sense of Human."

Harry Moskos, Editor
The Knoxville News-Sentinel

PREFACE

We all have moments in our lives which, in looking back, we see as a kind of Damascus Road experience. Times when we see the light. Or maybe just the entrance to the right tunnel.

It happened to me one afternoon in the early '70s when I caught myself sitting in our den talking to a middle-aged Lhasa apso with laser breath, as together we watched a man fall in love with his plastic-surgeoned-beyond-recognition sister on "Days of Our Lives."

Suddenly Knuckles looked at me out of the corner of his eye as if to say, "What are two intelligent beings doing sitting here in God's great and wonderful world watching this stuff?"

I needed liberating. Knuckles knew it, and I knew it.

I tried burning my bra, but the dadgum thing was polyester, so it just basically melted. I signed up for an Outward Bound freedom climb, but on the eve of my great adventure our youngest child woke up with spots and threw up all over my backpack. I tried tennis. For a while I thought I had found IT after I signed up for a course in Chinese brush painting at the YWCA, but the teacher kept having to ask me, "Vhat ess dis?" and I got the message.

In 1974 I swapped my TV Guide, my carabiners, my tennis elbow and my boar's hair paintbrush for an industrial strength dictionary, a swivel chair and a short course on how to change ribbons in a typewriter. After a couple of lucky breaks, I began my writing career as a columnist for The Charlotte Observer. With their good editors and patient, forgiving readers, I learned the ropes, so to speak. The first time a reader wrote a scathing letter taking me to task for something I had said, it got me so upset I wrote a six-page letter back explaining, defending and elaborating on just how misunderstood I had been. I asked Bob Ashley, then features editor at The Observer, to read my masterpiece, hoping — no, expecting! — him to be impressed with the way I handled an angry reader.

After he read my letter, he called me into his office, shut the door and gave me some advice I have never forgotten: "Ina," he said, "you had your chance. Every day your words are thrown up on people's front porches, and if they are interested enough to write you back, don't insult them by saying it all again in a letter. Besides. You know what? They may be right!"

I have been "throwing up" words in newspapers for over 20 years now. Without getting too mushy here, I think the best thing going for me has been my family and my readers. For years the kids were oblivious to the fact that they were being used as characters in my little nonfiction plots. Like most children, they paid no attention to what their mother was saying. Our son once told his teacher at school when asked if his mother worked that, yes, ma'am, she did. She sold Avon.

Maybe that's what I have been doing: landing on people's porches every morning, "selling" an idea, a story, a piece of information, an opinion. I can't help but think of something E.B. White — not an Avon pusher, but a best-seller of words — said about his writing: "I am constantly amazed that people will actually pay money to read what I think."

Well, I am sure no E.B. White, but if you're reading this, it means you have paid good money to read what I think. I hope it will be worth it to you. If not, write me. Because you know what?
You may be right.

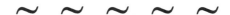

My mama taught me to clean up my own messes and put things where they belong — but she was mostly talking about toys. Hard as I try, there would have been a lot more messy typos and misplaced commas had it not been for long-suffering copyreaders like News-Sentinel columnist Sam Venable, retired features writer Christine Anderson and Margaret Dickson, retired children's librarian at Lawson McGhee Library. The paper dolls on Martin Gehring's cover look a lot better than any I ever cut out, and Miles Cary's camera did not break, as I thought it surely would, after he took my picture in the graveyard. That is a tombstone I am hugging, if you will notice. Miles knows how I hate to have my picture taken, so it was kind of appropriate that I seek other-world spirits to help me "say cheese."

A special thanks to my friend, Susan Alexander, News-Sentinel public service director, who edited this project with patience and good humor, and to the folks at The News-Sentinel for making it possible. Working for Harry Moskos is a privilege, because he is the kind of editor who gives you encouragement and energy to do your best.

I. DEEP THOUGHTS AND SHALLOW CONCERNS

There's a lot of talk these days about being left-brained or right-brained and what it means in terms of who we are and how we approach life and its challenges. Phooey. Whether we are intuitive or deductive, whether we have type A or type B personalities, whether we like our watermelon cut into wedges or smashed open on the sidewalk — when the shadows fall and the evening comes, we all want the same things. Fear the same things.

And, I'm sure, we all laugh at the same things. ·

Some of our concerns are deep and dark and take our breath away. Some are secret, silly hang-ups, and we would be embarrassed if others knew how much they bother us.

That's the only thing that makes me brave enough to 'fess up. Because I really believe that, way down deep, we all have the same basic concerns and questions.

And quirks.

A PRAYER
FOR CHILDREN

One Thanksgiving several years ago, I wrote a prayer for children as my column offering for The Charlotte Observer, where I was then writing three columns a week.

It was a very personal piece.

Somebody once said that a writer and a spider are to be pitied above all others because they both hang by a thread spun out of their own guts. I don't know about the pity part, but sometimes the things we feel the strongest are the hardest to articulate.

I got lucky that Thanksgiving, not because what I wrote was any great shakes as poetry, but because so many people in this world are concerned about its children.

What I wanted to say was that when we talk about loving kids and wanting the world to be good for them, we really are talking about two kinds of children.

3

There are ours. The ones we tuck in at night. The ones we once were, the ones we see skipping up and down the sidewalks in the neighborhood.

Then there are theirs. The others. Kids we might never see, who have no names we know. Children who are so disenfranchised by societies and governments, systems and politics that they come and go with hardly a notice from anybody.

The poem has since been used in schools and churches all over the country. I probably get two calls a week from people about it. It was read during UNICEF's World Summit for Children, has been reproduced in religious magazines and educational journals as well as by human service and advocacy groups and is being used by the Children's Defense Fund in its literature. It is the closing piece in Marian Wright Edleman's best-selling book, "The Measure of Our Success." It has been read three times on national television, been reprinted in a host of editorial columns throughout the country and even found its way into a segment on one of the soap operas. A friend of mine calls it "the poem that will not die." What I hope is that the concern it expresses will never die, because when that happens, we will no longer be *human* beings.

A PRAYER FOR CHILDREN

We pray for children
  who put chocolate fingers everywhere,
  who like to be tickled,
  who stomp in puddles and ruin their new pants,
  who sneak Popsicles before supper,
  who erase holes in math workbooks,
  who can never find their shoes.
And we pray for those
  who stare at photographers from behind barbed wire,
  who've never squeaked across the floor in new sneakers,
  who never "counted potatoes,"
  who are born in places we wouldn't be caught dead,
  who never go to the circus,
  who live in an X-rated world.
We pray for children
  who bring us sticky kisses and fistfuls of dandelions,
  who sleep with the dog and bury goldfish,

who hug us in a hurry and forget their lunch money,
who cover themselves with Band-Aids and sing off-key,
who squeeze toothpaste all over the sink,
who slurp their soup.
And we pray for those
 who never get dessert,
 who watch their parents watch them die,
 who have no safe blanket to drag behind,
 who can't find any bread to steal,
 who don't have any rooms to clean up,
 whose pictures aren't on anybody's dresser,
 whose monsters are real.
We pray for children
 who spend all their allowance before Tuesday,
 who throw tantrums in the grocery store
 and pick at their food,
 who like ghost stories,
 who shove dirty clothes under the bed
 and never rinse out the tub,
 who get visits from the tooth fairy,
 who don't like to be kissed in front of the car pool,
 who squirm in church and scream in the phone,
 whose tears we sometimes laugh at
 and whose smiles can make us cry.
And we pray for those
 whose nightmares come in the daytime,
 who will eat anything,
 who have never seen a dentist,
 who aren't spoiled by anybody,
 who go to bed hungry and cry themselves to sleep,
 who live and move, but have no being.
We pray for children
who want to be carried
and for those who must.
For those we never give up on,
and for those who don't get a chance.
For those we smother,
and for those who will grab the hand of anybody
kind enough to offer.

BATHING BEAUTY

My problems with swimsuits started way back when I was 7 or 8 and my mama took me aside, looked deep into my eyes and said, "The time has come for you to stop wearing your brothers' bathing suits."

Now you have to remember, this was a long, long time ago, and I was a very skinny kid.

Back then, the birds and the bees didn't start flying around in a kid's head until late in life. Like when you got really old. Say, maybe 15 or 16. Today's 8-year-olds are already blow-drying their hair and wearing lace underwear.

But this is now, and that was then.

I hadn't a clue as to what my mother was talking about.

At 8, I was allergic to lace, to frills, to

dresses, to ribbons, and to anything that had to do with hair, jewels, fingernails and Sunday shoes. Well, make that shoes, period. Any kind. My philosophy was that if God had meant for us to wear shoes, he would have come up with something better than patent leather or leather.

Cleanliness — like godliness, good manners and clothes that itched — belonged in the adult world, and I stayed away from adults and their world as much as possible . . . mealtimes and lightning storms being the only exceptions I can think of right off.

Especially during the good ol' summertime when my four brothers and sisters and I piled into our parents' station wagon (with real wooden sides) the day after school ended and headed for the beach, where we stayed the whole summer in the family compound with dozens of cousins, most of them boys.

Up until that fateful conversation with my mother, all I wore, all summer long, were my brothers' hand-me-down trunks. No top. No shoes. No socks. We didn't even change after we got wet. Sticky, sandy, smelly clothes only matter to sissies and old people. Real children don't give a hoot.

It came as a shock to learn that I had to start dressing like a girl. It was embarrassing.

My mother took me shopping, and we came home with my first all-new, all-girl bathing suit. What's worse, she threw away all my brothers' ratty, wonderful trunks and made me actually wear the thing. It was so awful looking I seriously considered giving up swimming that summer.

I even thought about giving up appearing in public ever again.

My brothers' bathing suits had all been comfortable and sensible. Baggy, navy blue ones with drawstrings. Or yellow with white stripes and elastic at the waist. My favorite ones were green with red sailboats all over them.

Girls' bathing suits were ridiculous looking.

You had to go into contortions to get into them, or out of them. You could hang yourself just trying to go to the bathroom.

They pooched out and made your skin dent in where the straps crossed. They rode up in the back and fell down in the front.

They had skirts with matching panties. Whoever thought that up was sick, sick, sick.

My brothers called me Frankenst-ina that summer because every time they sang "I see London, I see France, I see someone's underpants," I took a poke at one of them and usually ended up with a new scar somewhere on my person.

Ever since that summer, I've had problems with bathing suits.

Either there was not enough of me to fill in all the pooches and bulges, or there was not enough bathing suit to suit my parents.

Back in college, before stretch marks and middle age, the ones I liked often had price tags bigger than the suit itself.

These days, I've got other problems. Forget style. Forget price.

I have to find a suit that (1) has enough material to cover all unsightly parts, but (2) not so much that if I get wet, I go to the bottom like a lead balloon. Something between a G-string and a circus tent.

It really hurts my feelings when I find one that fits, only to discover there's not that much difference between the numbers on the price tag and the numbers on the size.

Each year, Sports Illustrated sells millions of copies of its swimsuit issue. You'd think they'd find one bathing suit that I could wear without getting arrested.

The magazine is NOT about swimsuits. It's about what's in them, and there's not much. In fact, I was about the size of those models when my mother and I had the little talk that turned me into a girl.

ANIMAL PROTECTION OR RELIGIOUS FREEDOM?

Whenever our family gets together with great aunts, cousins, old-timers, the conversation sooner or later turns to Aunt Ine and her hog-killing ritual.

Until her death when she was almost 90, every fall — that time of year when trees turn blood red and the spice of life and death hangs in the air — she took charge of this long tradition in rural American farm life.

I never actually saw her in the rubber apron and hip boots, her corn-fattened hogs pegged out on the line to dry. The family stories get told in that faraway voice of memory that mixes fact and fiction, but each version makes the same point: Here was a woman never without her lace handkerchief, whose house smelled of rose hips and peppermint, who never uttered a bad word in

her life, yet was known far and wide as the best butcher in
Scotland County, N.C.

The stories were spellbinding, but, to tell you the truth, I
always felt a little sick. I never let on to anyone that Ine came off,
to me at least, as slightly crazy.

I do remember my grandfather killing chickens. I watched
him do it, and they really did run around after their heads had
been cut off. I laughed aloud because it helped me not think about
what I was actually seeing.

As upsetting as these farm-family traditions were, I never
made the connection between hog butchering and the sausage we
ate with pancakes at the beach; between my grandfather and his
ax and the drumstick on my plate at Sunday dinner. It would be
some 40 years later that I decide to become a vegetarian, and, even
then, it is as much for health reasons as humanitarian.

Slaughtering animals is an integral part of rural America,
right up there with quilting parties and church socials. So is
hunting and fishing. My brothers seemed to walk differently, taller
somehow, after they came home with a kill. A dead duck or a dead
deer, if they were lucky, was a ticket to manhood.

My father did not think it fitting that I go with him, my
brothers and boy-cousins, although I begged.

He was surprised to learn that, at the ripe old age of 8, I could
put a live crab on a hook without squealing "ooweee goowee" like a
real girl, and it earned me an invitation to go deep-sea fishing with
him.

My rite of passage came when I pulled in a fish that had
swallowed the hook. I can still remember the shame, mixed with
an eerie fascination: the fish squirming in my hands as I pulled out
its insides, then watching it flip flop across the slimy deck until it
lay still.

The Supreme Court of the United States ruled in favor of the
Church of the Lukumi Babalu Aye and their arguments against a
1987 city ordinance in Miami which made illegal the killing of
animals in religious rituals.

The church is a Santeria congregation for whom the sacrifice
of animals is a sacred act, a religious practice that goes back to
Cain and Abel. Not only in Judaism and Islam, but all ancient
religions, animal sacrifices have been a symbol for devotion,

purification and blessing.

Santeria leaders assure animal-rights activists the killings are done in a humane way. The meat is eaten in a sacred meal, with leftovers given to homeless shelters.

"You can buy Chicken McNuggets in Hialeah," Jorge Duarte told a Time magazine reporter in defense of his church, "but you can't kill a chicken for religious reasons."

Most mainstream denominations spoke in support of the Church of the Lukumi Babalu Aye. Their concern was that government is getting too close to preventing religious freedom.

Courts have outlawed Mormon polygamy, Pentecostal snake-handling, and the use of mescaline in Native American religious rites. Should animal sacrifice be illegal?

And is there a relationship somewhere between the devout Santeria's right to sacrifice a chicken and our right to slaughter hogs in the backyard, then brag about how well we do it? To count animals we've shot or hooked as a kind of trophy?

Tough call.

Think about this the next time you pass the perfume tester trays at the mall. Some perfumes are made of animal "parts." Four common ones are: (1) ambergris, digested by sperm whales; (2) civet, a thick yellowish secretion of the anal gland of cats in Africa and Asia; (3) musk, a granular substance found in pouches on the musk deer of Asia; and (4) castoreum, which comes from beavers.

Kind of makes you want to stick to baby powder, huh?

COLOR ME CORNFLOWER

Roy G. Biv is dead.

You remember Roy, don't you? All we had to do in science class was to think of him and out popped the names of all the colors in the visible spectrum: red, orange, yellow, green, blue, indigo and violet.

Binney & Smith Co., makers of Crayola crayons, was the first to start hammering nails in Biv's coffin. First they stopped making green-blue, violet-blue and six other basic crayon colors and replaced them with newfangled colors like "cerulean frost," "twilight lavender" and "jungle green."

It was a sad day for the coloring book crowd. No longer could you decide for yourself whether the twilight in your picture was to be lavender or one of the other chewed-up crayons in your pack; and anyone who says a jungle is just one shade of green has never been outside of the think tank.

But things are getting even more complicated.

Now Roy G. Biv is taking a beating in the clothing industry. Catalogs make great bedtime reading, but if you ever actually order from them, you have to wing it when it comes to choosing colors.

Very few things are named after Roy G. Biv.

White is no longer pure and simple, and off-white is a rainbow unto itself. (What, pray tell, is the difference between "snow" and "virgin," when it comes to white? Unless Snow White wasn't a virgin, which means that not only is Madison Avenue messing with our crayons, now they are rewriting fairy tales. Isn't it enough that they bumped off Biv and the stork? Is Walt Disney next?)

Catalogs have a parade of colors you never heard of and, even after you hear of them, you're still color-blind.

In the off-white department, there is natural, sand, cream, nude, bone, stone, clay, tumbleweed, sahara, sagebrush, citron, champagne, wheat, putty, vanilla, oatmeal, thatch and flax.

There are other real brain-teasers like arugula, bottle, himalaya, planet and tuscan — all of which, by the way, are greens.

There's the patriotic trio: cinnabar, chamois, and framboise. Betsy Ross would have never believed it.

In the L.L. Bean catalogs, green is "cactus" and "hunter," and anything other than underwear white is called "oatmeal." J. Crew, for some reason I haven't figured out, is into one-syllable colors: surf, leaf, punch, reed, beet, spice. Talbots does a lot in blush and blossom.

The Tweeds catalog of colors reads like a new earth-tone religion: herbier, eternal, zodiac, solar, calcium, stellar, ozone and something called aurora . . . but if you ever see that color on the horizon, you'd better get out the prayer book.

Sometimes, it's hard to tell whether you are filling out an order for a new wardrobe or inventing a new recipe. Cocoa. Sangria. Grapefruit. Tabasco. Granny Smith. Popsicle. Mustard.

I don't know what you'd look like if you mixed all these up in a Sunday outfit, but I know what you'd feel like if you did it at the dinner table:

Pepto-Bismol.

Which, according to my husband, is exactly the color on the walls of our dining room. The name on the paint can said "watermelon."

With watermelon and Pepto-Bismol, at least what you see is what you get. With a color like "honey" — it's pot luck.

Is that as in sourwood or Sue Bee?

Are "peaches" red-ripe or green?

Is burnt sienna different from unburnt sienna, and has anybody ever seen an umber, rare or well-done?

"Atmosphere" is — surprise! — purple. Is seafoam really gray-green, except maybe after an oil slick?

And what does "flesh" mean . . . for all God's children?

Shortly after Binney & Smith Co. did their number on those eight old favorites in the crayon box, people started protesting. There was the National Campaign to Save Lemon Yellow, The Raw Umber and Maize Preservation Society (RUMPS) and the Committee to Re-Establish All Your Old Norms (CRAYON).

I propose we catalog readers get organized. How about calling ourselves the Coalition to Label Order forms with Readily-identifiable, Objective Xamples (CLOROX).

Color me confused.

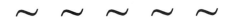

Color names aren't the only confusing things we face — spelling can be, too.

George Bernard Shaw said he knew at least four perfectly reasonable other ways to spell fish:

*1. **ghoti:** gh as in enough, o as in women, and ti as in nation.*

*2. **phusi:** ph as in physics, u as in busy, si as in pension.*

*3. **ffess:** ff as in off, e as in pretty, ss as in issue.*

*4. **ughyce:** ugh as in laugh, y as in hymn, ce as in ocean.*

THE POLITICS
OF PREJUDICE

Not long ago, someone asked a
question I'm still tossing around in
my head: "Who will be the next
group of people that it's OK to
hate?"

The hottest issue before church and civic
governments these days is whether people of
different sexual orientation are fully human
and deserve to be treated as such.

The church is wondering whether to give
them spiritual credibility; the government
must decide if they have legal status.

When this issue came before our local
county commissioners, church met state head
on and the sparks flew. It drew a crowd of
speakers, protesters, curious onlookers and
radicals from both ends of the spectrum.

Virtually everyone who spoke in favor of
not giving gays and lesbians legal status said
they were doing so out of obedience to the

words and teachings of Jesus Christ. That is, of course, the same rationale behind discrimination of blacks, women, Jews, Catholics, Germans, Japanese, native Americans and all the others we have allowed ourselves to hate in the name of God and country over the years.

At that meeting, Resolution R-93-3-121, which denies legal status to gays, lesbians and bisexuals, passed with 14 commissioners in favor, two against, two abstentions. One commissioner was absent. The county I live in is now on record as opposing gay rights and sent a message to our elected officials in Washington "to actively oppose legislation to include homosexuals or bisexuals in the Civil Rights Act of 1964."

Many disturbing things were said and done at the meeting, but I want to tell you about a little scene I witnessed as I stood in back, watching and listening. Sitting in front of me was a group that had been bused in to support the resolution. Each carried a large Bible in his or her hands and from time to time would wave it in the air. Judging from conversations I overheard, they came from a church outside the county, one of several, I understand, whose members had come by the busloads in response to a call to arms by a local "Christian" radio station.

I heard several of these radio pitches, the gist of which was to encourage "Bible-believing Christians" to go to the county commissioners' meeting and oppose the work of the devil, now cleverly disguising himself in the form of child-molesting, disease-carrying perverts who are an abomination, a threat to society because they are soliciting members in classrooms and the military, and a threat to the future of the human race because they can't procreate.

Anyway, the group in front of me believe all this very deeply and were there to speak up.

And speak up they did.

Whenever anyone approached the microphone to oppose the resolution, they would punch each other and make some snide remark. For instance: One gay man, speaking on the right of all Americans to be treated equally — "with liberty and justice for all" — said he had fought for this basic principle as a member of the military, having served and been disabled in Vietnam.

One of the "religious" guys on the row in front whispered to his buddy, "You are disabled all right." . . . chuckle, chuckle.

When a woman speaking against the resolution stated her occupation as a professional in waste management, another man in the group said, "Yeah, and you are a piece of garbage."

There were jabs and jokes, rolling of the eyes and snickers — be it over a woman in pants or a man with a soft voice or a minister from a different religious perspective.

When the resolution passed, the group turned to one another, lifted their fists and their Bibles, and pronounced another victory for goodness and truth. One of them turned to the crowd, raised his hands and said, "All you people need to just go home and ask forgiveness for your sins."

Which I did.

I asked God to forgive me for not speaking up to people who abuse the Bible by hiding their hate behind it.

But I also told God he'd better be glad I hadn't opened my mouth. I would have gotten angry and probably ugly . . . which, as we should all know by now, doesn't accomplish anything.

"Everyone lives in earthquake zones; the reality we know is always shaky." — Stephen Dobyns in "After Shocks / New Escapes."

TO BE OR
KNOT TO BE

There are, I have decided, two kinds of women in this world: Those who can wear scarves. And those who cannot.

I cannot.

Don't ask me if it's a genetic thing, a matter of training or some kind of phobia.

Every once in a while, I decide to try again, that it's silly to have this thing about scarves and surely if I just tie it right, I, too, can look like the saleslady who sold it to me.

"It makes the outfit," they always say.

But scarves make me crazy.

They come alive, like snakes wrapped around my neck. The knot gets loose, or the folds come unfolded, or everything switches around to the back.

I end up looking like I'm wearing a neck brace.

On the street other women swish along

with their $35 scarves looped to the side, one end tossed casually over the shoulder, the other neat and sassy down the front, and I go home full of hope.

But the only way it would work on me is to use a staple gun and avoid turning my head.

When I wear a scarf I look like I'm getting ready to hold up a bank. Or scrub for surgery.

My mother, who is really into scarves, thinks I just don't spend enough time getting myself together in the morning. She gave me three scarves for Christmas and a scarf clip for my birthday.

So, once again, I got out the "100 Ways To Tie a Scarf" book she gave me last year, set the alarm to allow a few extra hours to dress and gave it one more try.

By the time I got to work, the scarf clip had fallen down on the job, and my supposedly scarf "rose" (pages 4-6 in the book) had grown so big it looked like a paisley goiter.

For lunch, I had scarf tails dipped in Lunch Box gumbo.

Back in the office, I almost strangled myself when I leaned over and got caught in the bottom file cabinet.

I noticed people sort of tilted their heads when they talked to me, like something was offsides.

By late afternoon, my whole outfit had made a 180-degree turn. Everything was in place — even the blasted scarf.

The only problem was my head was on the wrong side of my body.

I've even tried to secure scarves on blouses that have shoulder loops, but by the time I get out the door and halfway to work, I look like something off "Bonanza" that just got roped.

Don't even suggest I use scarves to add a dash of color to my waist. The less attention I draw to my waist, the better. Besides, anything tied around my waist gets a real workout holding everything in; and if you've ever tried to get a tight knot out of a silk scarf, you won't give it such a big job ever again.

I finally put all my scarves in a shoebox and mailed them to my mother, but guess what? She never gives up. She sent me a red plaid cape.

"It's the family tartan," she said.

Now I look like a cross between Mother Goose and a bagpipe.

DIAL 0 FOR OUT-OF-IT

At 30, you lose your waist.
At 40, your eyesight.
At 50, your mind.
How do I know? Let me count the ways.

It all started the other day when I couldn't remember my phone number.

I was trying to call home to tell my husband I was running late. Very late.

Fifteen minutes after I was supposed to be at home, dressed and with a potluck dish in hand, ready for him to pick me up for a church supper, I was standing in the rain at a pay phone on the interstate, trying to call home and tell him to go without me and I'd meet him there.

It was no use. I couldn't remember our phone number, and I couldn't look it up in the phone book because the print was too tiny.

All the way home, my heart kept pace

with the windshield wipers. This was serious.

Swish swish swish.

Thump thump thump.

638-27 . . . 368-620 . . . 637-83 . . .

"It's no good," I cried as 18-wheelers threw mud and gunk all over my car, making me feel even more weak and helpless. "I'm a grown woman, and I don't know my own phone number."

We'd had a rule in my house when the children were little.

A thousand years ago.

They weren't allowed to go off by themselves until they passed the "Phone Number Test," and here I was, a grown woman on I-40 in practically a hurricane, without a clue as to whether it was 6-3-7 . . . 3-7-6 . . .

Or what came next.

Swish swish swish.

Thump thump thump.

I've always been good at remembering numbers. I make a game of it. Like when I learned my very first phone number, back in that other lifetime.

"Mr. Three," I told myself, "ate two four-sevens."

That was 45 years ago. Those numbers are still floating around in gray matter.

But what matters is my phone number now, and it was gone.

The more I thought about it — *swish swish swish, thump thump thump* — the more depressed I got.

I decided to look for other signs of senility.

All the way home, I recited Social Security numbers, birth dates, multiplication facts and how many days hath September, April, June and all the rest.

It made me feel better that those numbers still clung onto my frontal lobe. Why had my phone number given up?

A month ago, to the day, I had turned 51. Already I was on my third pair of bifocals. Somehow I hadn't expected my mind to go as quickly.

Just last week, after going through the drive-in teller at the bank, I forgot to give them back the plastic tube that sends out the money. . .

Swish swish swish.

Thump thump thump.

. . . two blocks down the road after cashing a check, I'd looked over at this strange jar thing on the seat beside me, and it took a minute to realize what it was.

And several weeks ago I stopped off at Mrs. Winner's to get some chicken to take my family for supper. I'd forgotten I didn't have any cash, but that was OK. They let me write a check. When I got home, I set the table, even lit a candle.

Guess what? No chicken. I'd driven off without it.

Swish swish.

Thump thump.

What was happening to me? There on the rainy interstate, my whole life seemed to pass before my eyes. The only detail left out was my correct and present phone number.

By the time I got home, my brain was soaking wet. Flying into the kitchen, I slapped a row of canned pears on a plate of lettuce, plopped a cherry on top to make it looked well-planned and (after reading my phone number off the dial face) raced into the den and wheezed to my husband that I was ready.

"For what?" he asked.

"The church supper!"

"What church supper?"

> *How do you spell a sneeze? We've all heard a thousand — but is it really ah-choo? Or is it more like arghrughcskxoo? Hahgggjhoo? Igmhghadjiii? Cheeewzzz?*
>
> *Gesundheit isn't really German for "Get your germs off me." It's German for "Long may you live." Pope Gregory the Great supposedly started this blessing of the sneeze during his reign when a plague hit Rome.*
>
> *Why did they say it in German? Because "Bless you" in Latin is "Pax!" With a word like "Pax!" after every sneeze in a pollen sneezing fit, it would be hard to tell who was sneezing and who was blessing.*

DESIGNER GENES

You know those great-looking new spring clothes in the magazines? Well, don't get your hopes up. Especially if you weigh more than a bread box and have normal body parts.

In a way, it's false advertising to model clothes you and I are supposed to buy on somebody who has nothing that pooches out except lips.

The other morning I came to breakfast in a new outfit. After all, it's spring. Time to shed the old cocoon. Time for a fresh look.

But it was my daughter who got fresh. She laughed so hard she spit chocolate milk all down the front of the newspaper.

"Mom," she said, "you can't go out looking like that. You have nice clothes in your closet. What makes you put on something like that?"

Wonder where she heard that lecture before? This time the shoe was on the other foot.

But it wasn't shoes that had her in stitches. It was boots.

"Fashion boots," the salesperson had called them. "They will look darling with your stirrup pants, a little T-top, then finish it off with some really fun earrings . . ."

I didn't have any stirrup pants, and I'd never thought of earrings as being much more than things you stick in your lobes — silver or gold on weekdays, pearls on Sunday.

So after I paid for the boots, I trotted off to the stirrup and ear departments.

I was really fixed up: Fashion boots. Stirrup pants with tiny glow-in-the-dark dots on them. A medium T-top (I would've been arrested in anything smaller). And the things clipped to my ears weren't earrings at all. They were little decks of cards.

I didn't look "darling" at all. I looked like a cross between a neo-Nazi and a Smurf.

It's not easy to be in style these days. There's a difference between how clothes look on runway models and people who live in California — and how they look on a person who eats daily from the five food groups and has some sense of pride.

Especially if they are over 10 and it's not Halloween.

Why can't designers take women the way God made us? Instead, they add shoulders, subtract chests, drop waists, file toes into sharp points and make us walk on sticks.

They make sweaters big enough to slipcover Rhode Island and pants so tight you have to lie on the bed to get them on. Doctors get a lot of business from women who actually try to bend over in them.

Skirts these days have so many pleats and gathers, you end up looking like the Pillsbury Dough Boy in drag.

Blouses are so long and huge that if you tuck them in, you need pants a size larger for the fabric storage. If you belt them in, you look like an elephant after she's been to the Banana Republic.

I don't know which is worse: too little or too big.

The other day in the mall, I saw an outfit on display that I really liked. When I dissected it, I discovered it consisted of a sweater, a blouse, an open-necked undershirt, a knit undershirt and a turtleneck under-under-undershirt.

Plus a scarf.

There wasn't any room in there for a real live person.

And, if there had been, it would have had to be a very small, cold-natured Eskimo.

So I didn't buy it. Instead, I bought my boot-stirrup-earring outfit. I still don't know what went wrong. They were the right size. They were the right color.

It was, as a matter of fact, raining outside, so one could say it was a day made for boots.

How could something that looked so good in magazines be responsible for chocolate-coating the morning paper and kicking me in the ego?

But I can take a hint.

I took them off, put on my shirtwaist with the elastic belt, my navy cardigan and sensible shoes, then sent my daughter up to get herself dressed for school.

Guess what she wore.

The United States has an estimated 17 square feet of shopping center space per person. From 1960 to 1980, the number of shopping centers grew from 3,000 to 20,000.

TRAGEDY AND INSPIRATION

Our daughter is in the throes of deciding her major at college. When she was 6 years old, she had her whole life figured out. If you asked her what she wanted to be when she grew up, she could tell you right off:

"A cheerleader for the Dallas Cowboys or a missionary like Mother Teresa."

Now she's not so sure, and the time has come for some grown-up decisions. She's leaning toward English, "but what can you do with an English major?"

Everything.

She was home between exams this past weekend for a 35-pound "wash off" down in the laundry room and as much sleep as trips to the movies would allow.

Whenever we asked how exams went, she fell back on the sofa, put a pillow over her head, and moaned.

But you can tell by the way she talks about the poem she analyzed on the English exam that she's discovered the magic of words. She loves unlocking their secrets, traveling into other minds and hearts on someone else's wings.

"Why are all the good poems so sad?" she asked this weekend. "Are writers unhappy people?"

Her question took my breath away because I remember asking the same thing back when I was a sophomore in college. I've still not found the answer.

Within the past several months, I have read a hundred or so poems and essays written by young school children. Teachers and editors give me the benefit of the doubt sometimes and ask me to help judge writing contests of one kind or another. It's a tough job, as I am sure you can imagine.

And, to be frank, most of the good poems are full of angst — that wonderful catchall, English-major word that means despair, guilt, fear and other rainy-day feelings. Does that mean writers have a mind that glows best in the dark? An eye that sees farther in a windowless room?

Are happiness and good health really corrosives? Do they rust the connections between mind and art? Do tears work like cold water on a sleepy face, waking up the best in us?

If Sylvia Plath had been head cheerleader and president of her sorority, would she have had the time, the inclination — the know-how — to pioneer the black hole of the soul?

Robert Louis Stevenson discovered treasures a rosy-cheeked child is too busy to notice. If Milton had not watched the light fade, would he have seen so clearly the realities beyond? Within?

Can you be a visionary if you have 20-20 vision?

Great sonnets aren't written over champagne in a room full of well-wishers. They're written over a crumpled letter or a silent phone. Freedom is sweetest and dearest when seen through red glare and bombs bursting. The maple tree is most remarkable at its own funeral.

The most beautiful song is saved for the third act when love is betrayed or misplaced or done in, and every ballerina wants the part of the dying swan.

Are the cutting edges of creativity sharpened by pain? Would Coleridge be Coleridge without his demon drug? Was it cleverness

or craziness that made Poe so darkly brilliant? Fitzgerald. Plath.
Bronte. Angelou. Sarton. Donne. Dickinson. Dylan Thomas. So
many, it seems — their art chiseled out of hard lives. Misfits.
Malcontents. The desperate. The dispossessed.

The best sermons are about sin. Sunsets look better through
the lens than do sunrises.

Maybe creativity is one part talent and a thousand parts fear
or misery: Thoreau's obsession with solitude; Martin Luther's
wrestling match with the angels; Katherine Anne Porter's self-
inflicted poverty.

Are poets, then, like firewood? Is it rough weather that makes
them burn? One of the best-sellers of the mid-20th century was not
written by a "writer" but by a 14-year-old girl hiding in an attic.

Is it really, then, talent that makes art? Is it imagery and
form, style and flow that turns words into paintbrushes for readers
to use in filling in the lights and shadows on their own souls'
canvases? Or is it more likely a cell gone haywire? A shove into a
den of lions?

Or an empty place at the table?

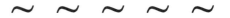

*Psychologists say they really don't know
very much about happiness. In its two volumes, the "Encyclopedia of Human Behavior:
Psychology, Psychiatry, and Human
Behavior" has no entry for "happiness," and
the word does not appear in the index.*

*Modern-day research indicates it is unre-
lated to money or physical beauty. They tell us
that whether a person finds happiness
depends on four psychological attitudes: (1)
emotional security; (2) a belief that life has
meaning; (3) a lack of cynicism; and (4) a
feeling of control over the good things that
happen.*

*Didn't Norman Vincent Peale and Mr.
Rogers figure all that out a while back?*

INFERNAL EQUINOX

Daylight saving time, they say, was invented by a man who cut off one end of his blanket and sewed it to the other to make it longer.

The problem is remembering which end to cut. Do we get ready for church in slow motion or fast forward? That is the question.

I know. I know. Spring forward. Fall back. But even simple things are hard to remember when getting children ready for Sunday school and church.

The changeover always takes place in that split second dividing Saturday and Sunday, while old people sleep and young people are just getting started.

Just for fun, let's look in on the Just-About-Any-Family the morning after that guy snipped off the wrong end of his blanket:

"Mom! We're outta milk!"

Just fix a piece of toast, dear, and, please,

go out to the car and get the dry cleaning.

"There's no bread either. And creep-head dropped a frozen blob of Minute Maid on the floor, so there's no juice."

Just pick it up and use it anyway.

"How can I? She spilled it last night. The dog's gotten in it. I think his mouth is stuck together . . ."

Well, just eat Oreos and milk.

"There's no milk."

JUST DRINK WATER. But, please, hurry up. Sunday school starts in 30 minutes.

"Mom! Have you seen my other white shoe? Mom! I can't find my shoe. Mom! Where are you, Mom?"

"Pipe down. Mom's in the shower, but not for long. There's no hot water. Heh. Heh. Heh. Wanna see how long it takes her to yell? Ten . . . nine . . . eight . . . ."

I'VE HAD IT!

"Blast off . . ."

Why do we have to play Eskimo every Sunday morning? It doesn't take other families 80 zillion gallons of steaming water to wash hair that wasn't dirty in the first place!

"Mom. Phone."

We could build our own lake with what comes out of our faucets . . .

"Mom. Telephone."

I figure we use six cups per strand of hair . . .

"Telephone, mother."

Hello. Yes, this is she. I'm fine, thank you. No, I don't need Arthur Murray dance lessons . . . but got any cemetery lots? Big enough to fit three very clean children, small enough for one shriveled-up old woman with blue lips? You do? Lovely. Send them right over. 'Bye. . . . Did you find the cleaning?

"What cleaning?"

The dry cleaning cleaning.

"Dad took your car to early church."

"Mom! Somebody stole my other white shoe. I can't find it."

Nobody stole your shoe. It's where you left it. Wear something else.

"What? The only other shoes in my closet are one white, two tennis shoes and my ski boots."

Wear the ski boots. God won't care. Start a trend.

"Mom! This isn't funny."

I'm not laughing.

"Can we go, Mom? We're going to be walking down the aisle during the sermon."

I might not live that long. I'll keel over from a heat stroke by the second hymn. All my summer dresses are in the attic. My only Sunday blouse went to church without me.

"Mom! I remember where my shoe is."

Good. Put them on and let's go.

"I can't."

I thought you said you found your shoe.

"No. I said I remembered where it is. It's at school . . ."

"Mom, did you fix the clocks?"

Yes. Uh. No. Did I?

"What time is it, Mom? Mom, what's that black stuff running down your face?"

Spring back? Fall forward? Or is it fall up, spring towards? Back spring? Fall over?

"Mom, your face is melting."

If I could get my hands on that numbskull with the blanket, I'd knock the daylights out of him.

"Why are your eyes crossed? Mom. Say something. Mom?"

~ ~ ~ ~ ~

Feel like yawning? Go ahead. Yawning is exhibit A on power-of-suggestion charts. Just thinking about it triggers a yawn.

Why not run your own experiment? Yawn real big, then wait a minute, and chances are someone who saw you will join you. Or give this to someone to read, and watch. People who get this far without giving in to a yawn really have a mind of their own, with higher-than-average immunities against the powers of suggestion. That's the nice way to put it.

Actually, they want to — but are just too darned stubborn.

A BAG LADY'S PLIGHT

Paper or plastic?"
I never know what to say. I realize I should take my groceries home in a think-green cloth bag, but I haven't figured out the logistics of getting two weeks' worth of supplies inside a rain forest tote. It would take a whole cotton field's worth of cloth to make it big enough.

But then I hate to think of how many trees get cut down or how much plastic floats in our rivers every time the Hughs family runs out of birdseed, mouthwash and Wheat Thins.

"Paper or plastic?"
Until lately, I'd never given it much thought. I try not to think at all in the grocery store. I just put my mind on automatic pilot and pray I'll get out of there with half my list, all my toes and enough money in the bank to cover the check.

It depresses me to think about all the fancy vacations, house repairs and college tuitions we could enjoy if we just didn't have to eat, scrub, drink, brush, scour, chew, gargle or polish.

Bringing home groceries not only takes large paychecks and large bags, it takes large muscles. Especially if you never go when you need *something*.

You wait until you need *everything*.

The Mother Hubbard approach.

So there I am in the checkout lane, a dozen bunches of things from the produce department getting smushed to death under a mountain of cans, boxes and jugs . . .

"Do you prefer paper or plastic?"

Have you ever noticed that all grocery stores fix it so the first place you come to is the produce department? Through the door, hang a right and there they are: all the breakables and squashables. By the time you get to the dog food — usually on the last aisle — you've got eggs on top of strawberries, underneath laundry powder, with frozen orange juice oozing all over loaves of bread flattened by pickle jars and shampoo bottles.

Plop 50 pounds of Gravy Train on top of all that and what do you get?

Grocery goulash. Hardly worth bagging at all.

"Ma'am. Do you want paper bags or plastic bags?"

I prefer boxes. After all, most of what we buy is square. Ram eight different kinds of cereal in a paper bag, and you've got 64 sharp corners poking holes and ripping it open.

Why eight? One of my early morning eaters is on a shredded wheat kick. Only one and only shredded wheat. Another read an article saying raisin bran fights heart disease. Her brother says raisins look like rabbit you-know-what, so he doesn't touch the stuff. Then there's my corn flake purist. He's eaten corn flakes since he was 7, and that was 48 years ago, so why should he change now? If it ain't broke, why fix it?

So. That's four different kinds, right? The other four were on special and will probably never get touched except by little bugs that bore past cardboard and wax paper like Marines at Dunkirk.

"So, lady. What'll it be? Paper or plastic?"

Plastic ones hook on your arm, so you can carry four at a time. It's kind of like wearing four 10-pound bracelets, so you're practically crawling by the time you reach the kitchen.

What they need are bags with wheels, like at the airport. That way you'd have a free hand to open the door when you got home. Nobody ever hears you kicking on the screen with your feet or ringing the doorbell with your nose.

Actually, you can hitch paper bags up on your hip and, after a lot of practice, learn to open the door with your chin, unless it's locked.

Which it usually is.

"Uh, lady, please. Paper or plastic? This is not a hard question."

But you know what they say about paper bags. That's where roaches make babies.

Paper bags make nice liners for trash cans, unless someone comes along and drops in a dripping grapefruit or half a carton of green milk. Then, when you go to take out the garbage, splat! There in the middle of the kitchen floor is the week in review.

"PAPER OR PLASTIC!!!!"

The pioneers didn't have so many decisions. Our foremothers drove to town in their non-station wagons, got a sack of flour, a few seeds, tucked them in an apron pocket, paid cash and that was that. Nowadays it takes a small train of oversized carts to get it all to the car.

And cash? I never carry around enough to pay for groceries.

Uh oh.

"OK, lady. This is it. Paper or plastic?"

"Neither. I forgot my checkbook."

HAIR TODAY, GONE TOMORROW

Nobody has ever called me a hysterical woman. Until now. But now, not only am I hysterical, if my passport were up to date, I would go live on another planet for about three months. Or ever how long it takes for hair to grow out.

It was not a wise decision to get a permanent.

"You would look bea-u-ti-ful," the hairdresser said, "with a little body wave on top. Come in sometime, and we'll fix you right up."

I don't look beautiful. I look like a fruit fly, and it wasn't a body wave, it was a frizz job, and I didn't get fixed up.

I got electrocuted.

Men won't understand. That may sound sexist, but there it is. My husband flat flunked the Understanding Test the moment he saw me.

He'd had plenty of time to think of some verse of scripture or some quote from Mr. Rogers that would make me feel better. We'd had an appointment to have our pictures taken for the church pictorial directory that afternoon. I called his office to say no way Jose. Not unless he could change the appointment to yesterday when, even though I didn't look beautiful, at least I looked human.

"He's in a meeting," his secretary told me, while I hid in the first phone booth I came to after leaving the beauty parlor.

"Get him," I practically sobbed into the receiver.

When I heard his voice, my throat got tight and my eyes stung.

I pictured him on the other end of the phone: nice face, nice physique, nice hair. Not the kind of man you'd pair up with a woman who looked like a cauliflower.

"My hair," I said, voice quivering. "It died. Cancel the pictures and come to the funeral."

There was a long silence.

Suddenly I realized that this was a scene straight out of one of those idiotic TV commercials that make women look like silly nits with nothing better to do than talk to the Tidy Bowl man or look for their reflections in a dinner plate. I could just see him after we hung up, turning to his colleagues with a Desi Arnez shrug, saying, "The wife is having problems with her hair."

"It's not worth getting so upset about," he said later when he saw it in person, but I could tell he was trying hard not to laugh. Easy for him to stay calm. His hair is thick and silver and always behaves. Mine has no color, no style, no curl.

Until now.

Now it has no color, no style and so much curl I could snip it off in little squares and sell it for Velcro.

My friends have been kind. "Wait a few days," they say. "It'll loosen up."

Only it hasn't.

Does vacuuming a shag carpet take out the curl?

Can you run a comb through a hook rug?

Ever tried to groom a roll of chicken wire?

I have washed, combed and used the hot brush so many times in the past 48 hours, I wouldn't be surprised to wake up tomorrow morning and find my hair on the pillow beside my head.

And I still look like a duckbill platypus.

There is no resemblance whatsoever between what's on the top of my head and "beautiful" — unless you are one of those people who makes art out of things most people throw in the trash. Andy Warhol is the only person I can think of who would like my hair, and he'd want to paint it and call it "Decadence IV23" or something like that.

Like hair balls in the shower drain or the fuzz in the dryer filter or a toothbrush that's been used to clean a thousand brass candlesticks.

That's what my hair looks like.

So don't anybody write me and tell me how lucky I am to have something, anything, on my head.

Or how lucky I am to have a husband willing to be seen in public holding hands with a Brillo pad.

Don't tell me that pretty is as pretty does. I could be a bloody angel and I'd still look like a cross between Woody Woodpecker and Big Bird.

And don't tell me beauty is only skin deep.

That has nothing to do with hair.

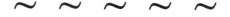

Each of more than 200 lashes on each of your eyes is shed every three to five months. Don't try to count them. You'll pluck yourself bald-eyed.

THINKING SMALL

People are always talking about the wonders of childhood — its innocence, the joy, the uncompli- cated world view.

When I was a child, I spoke like a child . . .

We all did.

Some of the words we spoke didn't make sense, but that didn't matter. Children don't have to make sense. I used to lie in bed at night saying aloud words that gradually modulated into yawns and carried me off in a wooden shoe, winking and blinking on a sea of crystal dew to a land where the moon talks.

Of course, it made no sense, but most of us can still quote those stories from childhood. To children, it is how words sound that give them meaning.

Words were toys back then: "Saskatch- ewan" . . . "kudzu" . . . "goose liver" . . .

"Tchaikovsky" . . .

Who cared what they meant? We just had fun trying them out, listening to how they worked up our throats and out into the silence around us. We were more into sound than sense.

Adults are supposed to make sense, to think things through.

Maybe that's why few adults "sleep like a baby" — the sleep of innocence that has a look all its own. When I can't sleep these days, it never occurs to me to call on Wynken and Blynken, and the only word games I play these days are crossword puzzles in the Sunday paper.

Words aren't toys anymore. They can even be dangerous. Sticks and stones only break bones, but words can kill.

You and I have to work hard to understand each other. It bothers us if somebody tells us we aren't making sense. We could get away with it as children, but as adults, we're held accountable.

Sounding good isn't enough anymore.

When I was a child, I understood like a child . . .

I knew money came from the bank, and you got all you wanted, plus a lollypop, if you just stood in line long enough. I understood that being old was wonderful because you got to drive and stay up late and tell people what to do.

I understood that only people who hated each other fought each other, and only people who loved each other went to church.

When I was a child, I thought like a child . . .

I thought babies were cooked in heaven like gingerbread people, and God walked by that heavenly bakery, poking each one of us in the middle, saying, "You're done . . . and you're done . . . and you're done." That's how come we had belly buttons. It's where God poked us.

I thought Santa Claus made it down every chimney in one night, and, for one happy morning, everybody everywhere had everything on their list.

I thought children all over the world ate too much on Thanksgiving and afterwards played Monopoly.

And never did it occur to me that there were people in the world who did not get a Valentine from anybody, ever.

If I had known, I would have been sad. But not for long.

When I was a child, my prayers floated up to heaven just like there was no roof, and I sat in the pew on Sunday morning and drew pictures during the sermon while my mother tickled my arm. I never had first — much less second or third — thoughts about anything I heard, or felt a single pang of sin or shame.

When I was a child, I thought people you loved never did anything to hurt you, and they always loved you back and they never went away.

I thought the world stopped at the end of my driveway and began with warm, pink sunlight smiling through white eyelet curtains.

But, when I became a man, I put away childish things.

There's only one thing worse, I suppose, than not ever having known the joys of childhood — the innocent, simple view of things. And that is not ever having given them up.

The world can't be run on make-believe.

We need to put away childish things.

But, if you really want to know the truth, sometimes I'd like to have them back.

II. FACES I WILL NEVER FORGET

The human mind is actually a little camera we carry around with us wherever we go. It moves through memory, through dreams, tags along strapped to our brains every waking moment . . . click-click-clicking away. Then, something we see years later or think about when we can't sleep at night will trigger the developing chemicals in those cerebral darkrooms, and a face will slowly come into focus again.

Too, there are people in our lives whose portraits hang in the foyer of our mind's eye. They are so much a part of who we are, they become like photographs in a locket we wear close to our hearts.

The more pictures we have in these scrapbooks and lockets, the luckier we are.

REACHING — FOR MISS MOON

O f all the once-upon-a-times I can remember, none is more memorable than the first day of school when I was in the ninth grade.

We'd moved that summer. The good-byes were little deaths, the hellos frightening and painful.

Everything was new: going to an all-girls school, catching the city bus to and from, wearing a uniform, and an English teacher in a wheelchair.

Miss Moon.

The name suited. She seemed cold, far away, mysterious. Dependable. Someone you could set your charts by.

"Eye-nah Jones!" (She's calling the roll that first day.)

I look up into those big, every-color eyes and forget my own name. If it had been a movie, they'd have played shark music.

I had decided that I was going to bury the name "Ina" and go back to the name I was called as a child.

Mackie.

It was a gift I was giving myself for having not committed suicide during the move.

So, there I am in the classroom that first day, looking up into those laser-like eyes and suddenly I could not speak.

Miss Moon's eyes didn't exactly undress you. I can't imagine she ever undressed anybody, or even had such thoughts. Her eyes pierced. A trite phrase, but there you have it. That's what they did.

"Eye-nah Jones!" she repeated, eyes just wide enough to send out little machetes that clipped my vocal cords. I just nodded.

From then on, forever and ever, I would be Ina.

Friday was Creative Writing Day, that ninth grade year. No holds barred. "Let go," Miss Moon said, but we wondered if she ever did.

"Be yourself."

Most of us had not a clue as to who we really were, and it was challenge enough just trying to play the part we'd been somehow assigned.

Sara Robinson was the Class Writer. On Fridays, Sara wrote stories in which phones "jangled." Connie Rucker, Most Popular, wrote about boys at dances and the things she didn't do. Marian Richardson, the Beauty Queen, got into a kind of serial about a famous actress named Suzanne. Only she pronounced it "SuzAHnn." And so on.

The only vacancy open for the New Girl was Class Clown. I wrote about the duckbill platypus. Or Chinese Siamese triplets named Yu Hoo, Me Too and Who Zit.

Each week my story was a gift I gave the class because, every Friday, Miss Moon herself read aloud each paper, and it was a memorable sight watching her upper lip curl over words like "platypus" and "zit."

She had the kind of voice that gave platypuses and zits stature just by the way she said them. She had the most commanding voice I have ever heard. It was a wonder her legs didn't just forget whatever it was that kept them resting under their plaid blankets and do what they were told.

Of course, her hair was white. She was born with it. I'm sure the doctor had come into her mama's hospital room and told her what a nice little white-headed baby girl she'd had.

That is, if Miss Moon had ever actually been a baby.

But it was her eyes that stopped any outright mischief dead in its tracks. Blinking to her was not a reflex activity. It was — as with everything she did — deliberate.

Each blink was a blink unto itself.

Like a frog's.

One Friday after English class, in a voice that sounded like our moving van turning in the gravel driveway, she told me she wanted to see me after school. I couldn't have gathered up enough spit to lick a stamp. My story that day — no holds barred, remember — had been about an amoeba that wanted a sex change operation.

School rules had it that we stood whenever a teacher entered the room. You'd think standing over Miss Moon would give you an advantage. Somehow, it made her seem even bigger. Like she encircled you from all sides.

Pierced and encircled that day after school, I got the shock of my life.

"Ina," she said, and there was no gravel in her voice, "you can make jokes with your life, or you can make something out of it. Life and the special talents we are born with are gifts, but a gift is nothing if you don't use it, and it's an insult to those who gave it to you. You can't spell and you don't always follow directions, and I can't read your handwriting, although I realize you try out a new one every Friday. But . . . "

Miss Moon was right. Life is a gift, and I did love writing those stories, and I loved the language she taught me to move around in.

Recently I went to a writers' conference in New Mexico. Each of us was asked to recall the person who had turned on the lights for us as writers. Every person there named a teacher.

I hope Miss Moon heard me call *her* name — as she once called mine.

PLAYING IT
BY EAR

I f I didn't know better, I'd have sworn "Dear Abby" was talking about my Uncle Hervey.

Tennessee made the headlines in Abby's column when a woman wrote about her husband's family and their tendency to crush ribs and deflate lungs when they hugged people hello.

The last time she went to visit, the woman told Abby, her mother-in-law hugged her with such enthusiasm it sprained her neck. Her husband once gave one of his Tennessee cousins such a hearty greeting, he broke three of the poor guy's ribs.

Sounds like some of my kinfolk.

My Uncle Hervey had a way of saying hello that made you see stars. His specialty wasn't ribs.

It was ears.

"Say hello to your Uncle Hervey!"

The first time I heard those words, I innocently padded over, looked up into the stratosphere (he was at least 12 feet tall) and did what I was told.

"Hello, Uncle Herv-OUCH!"

He didn't just tug or pinch ears.

He grabbed hold and twisted. Sometimes the lobe would end up on top when he finally let go, which he did only after he'd gone into painful detail in his deep scratchy voice about how he remembered when my daddy was my age and how I'd inherited his squinty-eyed smile.

We always knew which cousins had just come from saying hello to Uncle Hervey. They were very quiet, too busy swallowing baby tears to say anything — and they held their head funny, like they were trying to keep something from falling off.

But the ear twistings were a small price to pay for having an Uncle Hervey who owned the local railroad company and every visit would arrange for us to ride from Laurinburg to Hamlet, up with the engineer who let us blow the whistle every time we came to a crossing.

One summer at the beach, when we knew Uncle Hervey was coming, my brother Jimmy went down to the pier and bought out the supply of Bazooka bubble gum in the little Tootsie-Roll-style packs they used to come in, five wads for a nickel.

For days, we chewed and chewed until we got the sugar out and could work with the gum to design and mold a fake set of ears to fit our faces. It took lots of gum to come up with two that looked real.

And matched.

The night Uncle Hervey was due, we went Rock-Paper-Scissors to determine who would go first when time came to "Say hello to Uncle Hervey."

We figured that once he actually did what he'd been trying all these years to do — namely, unscrew an ear from some child's head — maybe he would be satisfied. Or at least get the hint.

One twist and he'd have a pink, flesh ear stuck to his fingers.

I suggested we really get even by having catsup in our hand so when we grabbed the side of our head after the first twist, we'd send blood gushing out, and Uncle Hervey would REALLY be sorry.

But my brother Bobby didn't think that was such a good idea. Especially since he was the Rock to three Papers and no Scissors.

Bobby went in, Uncle Hervey twisted, the Bazooka ear fell off, everybody laughed, and Bobby came out.

When my turn came to "Go say hello to Uncle Hervey," fate was not so kind. Before I'd taken two steps, my left Bazooka fell off. Uncle Hervey took one look at me, smiled his squinty-eyed smile, grabbed my naked left ear by the stem and wound it like a pocket watch.

As time passed and we got older, Uncle Hervey lost interest in our ears and took to knocking the wind out of my brothers with slaps on the back. We girls got something between a charley horse and a slug on the shoulder. Eventually, Uncle Hervey became too weak to slap or hug or even speak, and going in to say hello was something we dreaded, not because of a tug on the ear, but because of a tug on the heart.

My legacy from him after all these years is a squinty-eyed smile that's been recycled in varying degrees in my own three children; a stop-dead-in-your-tracks love of train whistles — and a left ear that is definitely larger than the other.

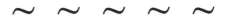

My favorite look-alike story is what happened to Charlie Chaplin when, unbeknownst to the judges, he entered a Charlie Chaplin look-alike contest in Monte Carlo.
He came in third.

MARK —
FOREVER YOUNG

I t has been more than 20 years since we saw Mark.
Then the other night we showed family movies — and there he was. Same teeth missing. Same cowlicks jutting out the top of his head like antlers on a small deer.

The first time I saw Mark, he was sitting on the front steps of our house in Norfolk, Va., talking to the birds. At least, that's what he said he was doing. There weren't any birds around that I could see, but when you are 3 years old, you don't actually need to have something around just to be able to talk to it.

"Wanna sit on the steps with me?" he asked in a voice so appealing it never occurred to me to step over him and take my groceries inside.

Pretty soon I was chirping right along with him.

Perhaps if I had known what was ahead

for all of us who came to love Mark, I would not have turned myself over to him so willingly. When he came by our house for a cookie, he not only got cookies, but all the Kool-Aid and conversation he wanted. Plus all the hugs he could stand.

One of those scenes in our family movies shows Mark coming piggyback across the lawn with my husband "giddy-upping" silently into the camera. We had no children yet, so it was Mark, you might say, who got that horse warmed up for the thousand rides to come.

I remember so well the day those pictures were taken and how Mark ended up grinning at us forever and ever from around a box of Christmas ornaments.

He and my husband had struck a deal: If Mark would help us decorate our tree, he could have a few branches off it to decorate and put in his room at home.

His folks told us later Mark kept his tree long after all the others in town had been stripped bare and pitched out. When you're 4 — and Mark turned 4 that winter — it doesn't have to be Christmas for you to enjoy popcorn and cranberries on the branches of a Scotch pine. Sometime later, he carried his tree out in the back of the garage and fixed a place for the birds to come "wait for each other."

That spring Mark grew so much his mother had to add strips of material to his overall straps to lower the hems. By summer, all his pants had patches on the knees, for Mark had discovered he could talk better to the birds if he got up in the trees with them.

By fall, we had moved to Washington, D.C., and kept up with Mark only through an occasional letter from friends.

Shortly before Christmas, we got a letter from Mark's family. Mark had leukemia.

When we brought in our tree that year, we cut off a little one from the top and put it in the room we were fixing up for our new baby.

By spring the news was worse, and one night we got a phone call from Mark's father. They were bringing him to the National Institutes of Health in nearby Bethesda, Md. We insisted they stay with us, and the next afternoon we sat staring at each other in our living room.

Then, jabbering in high-pitched make-believe, we rolled out

the sleeping bag and pulled open the sofa bed, like it was all some sort of game. Mark looked so different in his blue baseball cap he wore all the time because he had already lost most of his hair.

The cap always sat crooked on his head.

The doctors examined Mark and decided if he came to their hospital and lived in a room there and took their strong medicine that maybe — maybe — he would live a few months longer.

Mark's parents rolled up their sleeping bag and gathered up their son and took him home to his yard of trees and birds and his own room.

I don't remember when it happened, but I will never forget how.

When Mark's inappropriate but inevitable time came, his parents once again took him out of the hospital bed with its iron rails and away from the cold, static sounds of doctors being paged and brought him home.

He died early one morning as he lay in his own bed between his mother and father. The birds were just waking up.

Even after all these years, sometimes when I see a kid with a baseball cap on crooked or hear the birds waking up on an early spring morning, I think about Mark.

And I love him all over again.

MAKING BELIEVE
THE TRUTH

She was my best friend. So smart, so much fun to be with. But sometimes friends grow apart over the years, especially in friendships like ours. Her name was Verifrickus.

I don't know where such a name came from. I don't remember when she started coming to see me. I do, however, remember when she stopped.

We were driving home from a visit to my grandmother's, and I was lying across the backseat of the car with my feet sticking up in the window ledge, watching the world fly by.

It suddenly seemed a little babyish for a 6-year-old to have a friend nobody else could see or hear.

Or believe in.

So Verifrickus disappeared right then and there, just like the trees that flew out of sight past the car windows, like dancers making a quick, silent exit.

But I'll never forget her.

She used to sit at the dinner table and fish the cooked carrots off my plate, drop them into her napkin, then ask to be excused so she could flush them down the toilet.

She knew exactly where my brother's shins were under the table, and her aim was perfect.

Once she actually told my father to shut up. She said it very quietly, but he still heard.

She never, never did that again.

Through thick and thin, Verifrickus was there. I think about the night my little sister took a sip of some ammonia that had been carelessly stored in a 7-Up bottle. Her lips swelled, she screamed bloody murder and the doctor rushed over.

Verifrickus came and watched the whole thing with me from my hiding place on the back steps. The whole thing was my fault, I told my only friend. But God should know that just because you'd wished your baby sister would drop dead didn't mean you actually wanted her to die.

By far the most fun Verifrickus and I had together was when we would take my collection of little glass animals out in the garden in back of my house. We'd build villages for them out of sticks and acorns. If we were lucky, we sometimes found mushrooms that became a home for a ceramic squirrel or an umbrella for the frog with the chipped-off leg.

Verifrickus understood me, but people did not understand her.

Chuck Lambeth once caught me and Verifrickus playing make-believe, and he went off telling everyone he'd seen me talking to myself. If anybody had ever asked me why I wanted to go to heaven, I'd tell them it was because I knew Chuck Lambeth would not be there.

Once — just once — I tried to tell one of my friends about how important Verifrickus was and how I didn't care if she was real or not because it was fun to pretend.

The friend listened and acted as if she didn't think it was anything too awful, my confession. Later, I saw her standing by the water fountain telling what I said to a group of other kids. They were laughing.

It was a confusing lesson.

Real friends are supposed to stick by you.

In all of the bad things Verifrickus did — kicking my brother, sassing my father, even wetting the bed once — she never laughed at me.

Verifrickus never came back after that car trip home, when I watched the trees slip off into the night. But years later, I met some of her relatives.

One was named Ashley, and she lived in the closet behind the clothes in my own 3-year-old daughter's room. Another didn't really have a name, but he used to eat butter out of my refrigerator and let Popsicles melt on the sofa.

They, too, eventually flew off somewhere along the trip out of childhood, but I am sure that sometimes they are remembered — and thanked — for sticking by their special friend.

Sometimes the best magic of all is found inside your own head.

HORRORS IN THE BEST OF HOMES

From the outside, they looked like a Norman Rockwell family: Close-knit. Church-going. Civic-minded. He worked for the government. She was a homemaker. Their nine children were straight-A students. Little League and Girl Scouts.

The backbone of America.

But, behind closed doors, it was a different story.

A story so awful it became Their Secret, and anyone who bucked the system was drummed out of the family.

Mary was the seventh child.

For her, it started when she was 4 or 5.

She walked into the kitchen one morning in her pajamas and said something to her mother that made her mother mad. She grabbed Mary by the arm and gagged her.

Then she threw her into a hall closet,

turned out the lights and locked the door.

"I didn't understand what I had done," says Mary, "but I knew it was something awful. I was afraid to take off the gag. It might make her madder."

Mary spent all day in the closet.

"That night I heard the family eating dinner, talking as if nothing was wrong. They had forgotten me . . . but after supper my father came to the closet and opened the door. When he saw that I had wet my pajamas, he got so mad he beat me with an oar and put me back in the closet."

Mary stayed there all night, locked in the dark.

"The next morning, when my father saw that I had wet my pants again and had bled on the floor from where he had hit me — he hit me again."

And again. And again.

Until Mary was 14. Then suddenly the beatings stopped.

Now 28, Mary is struggling through the psychological garbage that is the cruel legacy passed from one generation of abused children to another.

"My mother kept lists of things I had done and would show it to my father when he got home from work. Losing a shoe, maybe. It could be anything. Or nothing. But it was always something."

Except for that first time, it was always her father who beat her, but her mother was there. Sometimes her mother sat and flipped through the pages of a magazine while her father beat her with the oar, or a chair, or his fists.

"I went through millions of different theories on why he was doing this, and they all boiled down to . . . well, it must be something I've done, or something I am."

Mary still has problems with the "why." Intellectually, she knows that for a 240-pound man to beat a 5-year-old makes no sense no matter what the child has done. Yet every beating was prefaced with the words, "I am doing this because you are bad" — and that imprint has left its mark on Mary long after the physical scars have healed.

"When I got older, there was a clear message that I 'should not have been a girl' — since most of the beatings were aimed at sexual areas. I also came to realize that my mother had been raised in an alcoholic family and my father had been abused as a child."

Mary is one among a growing number of children in our society whose monsters are real. In 1986, 2.2 million American children of all socio-economic levels were reported abused. Mary is one of those whose abuse was never reported.

It's contagious violence. Studies show that a third of all girls and two-thirds of all boys who grow up in abusive homes continue that violence in their own relationships. A hundred percent of San Quentin inmates reported suffering extreme physical abuses between the ages of 1 and 11.

"One of my older sisters tried once to intervene, and my father told her to 'butt out.' She left home the next day and never came back."

To her eternal credit, Mary decided to work through her pain. She decided she would not pass her abuse on to anyone else.

"I know that at least one of my sisters is abusing her own children."

After two and a half years of counseling with a trained minister, Mary has worked hard to heal wounds inflicted by her toxic parents.

"Someone once said that abuse leaves a child an emotional cripple. I know I can't change the past, but I hope soon to be able to walk away with, hopefully, a hardly noticeable limp."

To others who deal with similar problems, Mary has this advice — and warning:

"If you push your pain deep inside, it will multiply. You might say to yourself, 'I'll never do that to my kids,' . . . but if you don't deal with the pain, you pass it on to others no matter how strong your vow is."

SINGING AWAY
OUR SORROW

I t's never too late to sing.
That's a funny lesson to learn in the
middle of a funeral — especially when
you've never actually met the person
whose funeral it is.

But that's what I learned at my friend
Jackie McClary's father's funeral.

Jackie is a reporter for The News-
Sentinel, and for almost a year, our desks
were right across from each other. I don't
know how she would describe it, but some
friendships were just meant to be. The first
time I heard her laugh, I knew she was
somebody.

We have a lot in common, although I am
— ahem — a little older. Ten years, but who's
counting?

She and I are our own little support
group. Any working mom will know what I
mean. When Bryan, her 8-year-old, called to

say his brother was picking on him or that all the milk smells funny and should he drink it and, if not, what could he have for a snack — I could give her a knowing glance from across the aisle.

When my daughter was on her first road trip and called from some filling station phone in Florida to ask what it means when that little red light thing on the dashboard starts flashing — Jackie could give me a hang-in-there nod from the sidelines.

We share a lot of things: growing up in the South, a love of music, the same shoe size and microwave popcorn attacks about 4 every afternoon.

She'll laugh at my jokes even when they aren't funny, but she doesn't laugh when I ask her how to spell words anybody who has passed the fifth grade ought to know how to spell. She just spells them for me.

She's a singer who can sing.

I'm a singer who can't but does anyway.

We've been known to get off on old hymns, old hits — even old movie scores.

When I heard she was to sing on the radio as guest on a public radio fund raiser, I turned on all three radios in the house as loud as they'd go and stood in the hall to get the full effect. She was really something.

We both grew up in big families, and we both go to church every time the door opens, mainly because we want to but also because we both grew up in minister's families where nobody ever asked, "Are you going to church?"

Of course, we were.

Unless we had the bubonic plague, we were/are going to church.

She is Baptist. I am Presbyterian. But we memorized all the same verses and know all the same stories.

It was on a Sunday night that Jackie's father — the Rev. Richard Samuel Brown Sr. — died of heart failure. He'd been in poor health a while, but no matter how "prepared" we are, it's always a sock in the stomach.

Twenty-three years ago this fall, my father died of a heart attack.

I went to the Rev. Brown's funeral at the Bethel Missionary Baptist Church in Alcoa. Only they didn't call it a funeral. It was a

Homegoing. It began with a song, and it ended with a song. And, in between, there was crying and blessing, praying, clapping and giving thanks for a life that burned like a candle in the darkness.

There was a lot of music.

Maybe an unusual amount because music was an important part of the Brown family. Whether it was the choir singing or the organ playing or the congregation joining in, you could hear a constant, rhythmic pulse as people tapped their feet to the music.

It sounded like a gentle heartbeat.

As part of the service, Jackie and her brothers and sisters sang three of the Rev. Brown's favorite songs:

"Daddy loved to come in and see us sitting around, Mama playing the piano, and all of us singing. It was just about his favorite thing."

With that simple introduction, Jackie stepped back and the Brown children — now all grown with children of their own — sang for their father.

I never sang for my father.

His funeral was very different. Nobody tapped their feet. Nobody clapped their hands. Hardly anyone spoke above a whisper.

Sitting there during the Rev. Brown's Homegoing, I wondered why the funerals in my tradition are so controlled.

My father would have liked Jackie's singing.

What would have happened if I'd had the nerve twenty-three years ago to stand up and say, "One of his favorite things was to sit at the piano and play jazzed-up hymns. And one of my favorite things was to sit on the piano bench with him."

What if I'd played for him one last time?

It would have been fitting, especially if I'd done his version of "Beulah Land" or "Bringing in the Sheaves" that I learned from watching and listening to him.

Instead, at my father's funeral, we sang "For All The Saints Who From Their Labors Rest" and tried not to cry.

It's not a hymn you can tap your feet to.

So, like happens with friends, Jackie helped me out. Maybe, in a mysterious, complicated way, she helped us all.

Because when she sang for her father, she sang for mine, too.

And for all the saints who from their labors rest.

SKIING IS BELIEVING

Donna Clark not only came, saw and conquered the slopes at Snowshoe Mountain Resort. She saw the sun, the stars — and even a couple of moons.

"YEAH, I'M WITH THE KNOXVILLE GROUP," she yelled over the noise of the snowmakers. We'd ended up next to each other on our first ride on the chair lift during Ski School Lesson One.

". . . BUT I'M SCARED TO DEATH OF HEIGHTS AND I DON'T KNOW WHAT I'M DOING ON THIS THING. MY FRIEND JACKIE SAID THIS CLUB TRIP WAS THE BEST WAY TO LEARN TO SKI, SO HERE I AM. YOU'D THINK A GROWN WOMAN WITH HALF A BRAIN WOULD HAVE BETTER SENSE."

Her eyes got as big as saucers as we neared the top.

Moments later, she was seeing stars.

"OH, MY LORD!" she said, scooting on all fours, sideways, like a sand crab, trying to outrun the chair lift.

"DID YOU SEE THAT?" she asked, goggles knocked sideways and hair freshly frosted with landing-strip snow off the Skidder lift. "I DID EVERYTHING THE INSTRUCTOR SAID. . . BUT I FORGOT TO GET OFF!"

Donna was a fast study. A natural. She had the form of a real pro in her silky purple ski outfit. ("I BOUGHT IT FOR THE TRIP BECAUSE I JUST KNEW I WOULD LIKE IT AND WANT MY OWN STUFF.") And she quickly learned the right stance, the right moves, the right moment to slide forward and get off the lift.

The only thing she had real problems with was stopping.

Like the time she skied through two classes there on the beginner slope. First she knocked down an instructor, then scattered eight or 10 participants — some wide-eyed in amazement, others knocked clean off their skis without ever knowing what hit them.

"I CAN'T STOP!" she said in fair warning as she got closer and closer. "HEY, Y'ALL. I CAN'T STOP!"

If they had not had their backs to her, listening with rapt attention to their instructors, they might have noticed her before it was too late.

"I GUESS YOU COULD SAY I 'TOOK' THREE CLASSES AT ONCE," she said on the next trip up the lift.

After Lesson Two, Donna was ready for the big slopes. "NOTHING VENTURED, NOTHING GAINED, RIGHT?" she said as we plodded over to Powderidge, one of the "green" slopes recommended for beginners.

"TIME TO LIVE IN THE FAST LANE," she said as we high-fived each other before saying our prayers and pushing off on our first real run.

Then it was my turn to see stars.

"I CAN'T STOP!"

Recognizing that voice, I did a quick, just-learned J-turn to the side of the mountain and held my breath.

Zooooooooooooommmmmm.

She went by like a shooting star. I bet no person in the history of skiing has moved as fast in a snowplow wedge.

This time, she was lucky. People paid attention. Right and left, skiers parted, and Donna Clark of Pineville, Ky., took that hill like a pigeon-toed Olympian, never even slowing down until she hit the ropes that marked off the lift lines at the bottom of the hill.

They make those ropes, thank goodness, out of some kind of rubberband stuff that catches you, then hands you back all in one piece.

"BUT IT BROKE TWO OF MY FINGERNAILS," she yelled as we rode the lift to wherever it was going. Neither of us had brought our reading glasses, so we hadn't even tried to read the trail map. "I GUESS IT WAS NOT SUCH A GOOD IDEA TO GO GET FIBERGLASS FINGERNAILS RIGHT BEFORE COMING ON THIS TRIP. I'M MISSING TWO, AND I CAN FEEL THREE OF THEM LOOSE INSIDE MY GLOVES."

New skiers have a lot to learn. It came as a shock to learn that we had skied ourselves to the other side of Snowshoe, and all the lifts and all the slopes were now closed. So we had to take off our skis, walk up the hill past the Powderidge Condominiums and wait for the bus to take us back to our lodge.

That's when Donna Clark got mooned.

I never did ask Donna how old she was, but let's just say I know these guys weren't mooning me.

"OH-H-H-H MY-Y-Y-Y-Y STA-A-A-R-R-R-R-S," she said. "LOOK UP THERE IN THAT WINDOW. NO. DON'T LOOK. CAN YOU BELIEVE IT? DID YOU SEE IT? DON'T LOOK! ARE THEY STILL THERE? . . . HOW OLD ARE THEY?"

I allowed as how I didn't have a clue to the answer to that one. There wasn't much to go on.

By Lesson Three, Donna was a threat only to those who couldn't hear well.

"I never could get that stopping down," she confessed at the wine and cheese party the last night. "But I'm not going to let that slow me down. I can't wait to get back on skis again. I've been BITTEN BY THE BUG!"

THE HIDDEN WORLD OF JIMMY CLOVER

People in our neighborhood could set their watches by Jimmy Clover. Every afternoon at 4:30, up Providence Road and down Brook Road he came with head bowed in prayerlike concentration, hands cupped over his lips.

During the week, he came and went alone, but on Saturdays, people stopped raking leaves or pruning azaleas to watch — even listen.

Sometimes from a kitchen window came a wave, but, if Jimmy saw it, he never let on.

Nothing kept him from his concerts. They were never rained out. He never lost interest. No holiday cancellations. Not even the icy fingers of a dark January afternoon or the hot fists of August stopped him.

Always, he played his harmonica.

The fact that there was no harmonica

never seemed to matter or keep him from making his music.

Jimmy was a special person, an ageless child.

For him and 1.6 million other mentally retarded persons in this country, he'd been given a script he could not decode.

On Monday, Wednesday and Friday mornings, Jimmy Clover went to his job at a dry cleaner's. Carefully, and with a quiet dedication that should shame any of us who don't appreciate the gift of being able to do hard work, he put nonslip plastic covers on coat hangers.

Saturdays, he swept the driveway of the three-bedroom house where he lived with his sister and her family. Every Sunday night he walked up to the Presbyterian church on the corner to watch us shoot baskets or cook hamburgers.

Years later, when his sister's son turned 14, Jimmy Clover probably didn't figure out why his sister started planning special outings for the two of them on Sunday nights — which meant he couldn't go to youth fellowship with his nephew.

Like many mentally retarded adults, Jimmy resembled the people around him more than he differed from them. When one of us tossed him the ball those Sunday evenings in the churchyard, he tried harder than most to throw it back strong and straight. If he didn't smile and joke back when we clapped at his successes, it was, I suspect, because every part of him was busy soaking up the joy of the moment.

I once asked my father about his harmonica concerts, and he explained it this way: Jimmy Clover's ears and mind were not fine-tuned enough to read notes or even distinguish sounds, but his soul, too, needed to make music.

So he created his own.

Occasionally we made fun of Jimmy, I am ashamed to say. Behind his back. Never with the intent to be cruel, but, of course, it was.

To our parents' credit — for they set good examples — most of the time we looked after Jimmy with grave kindness and, at times, such tenderness that, if caught at it, we were embarrassed.

I'm sure all of us who knew him as kids think of Jimmy now and then. We'd be about his age now.

As it turned out, one of the girls in that church youth group had a retarded child herself years later. A boy.

Experts say that in any group of 10 friends, someone will have a mentally retarded person in their family.

I hope it gives her courage to remember Jimmy's music, but the jokes she made behind his back probably haunt her.

As mine do me.

There are so many whys about his life, but as for what his silent symphonies came to mean in the long run for a gang of neighborhood kids — you and I better hope we do as well with what we have.

THE LAUGHING MAN LIVES ON

Whenever I think of my father, I think of the Laughing Man. Like a character in a silent movie, his face comes in a quick close-up, without warning: eyes squinting in the sun, saying words I cannot hear.

It is June and we are at the beach.

The day school was out back then, our family would squeeze into an old green Buick with real wood sides and head for Wrightsville Beach, two-thirds of the way across North Carolina.

My mother had a theory about public rest rooms, so it was a long trip. Each of us had our own wet washrag in case we got carsick.

Which somebody always did.

When we finally got there, my brothers would haul in the suitcases, my little sister would be put on a pallet in the sun-room until mother could get the beds ready, and my father would come out in his one pair of shorts to "open the house."

I'd hold the ladder while he climbed up to undo the shutters all around.

He had big kneecaps.

The next day, Daddy would drive back to the city. We stayed all summer, and he came only for a few days every two weeks or so.

That's when he'd tell us about the Laughing Man.

His favorite meal was roast beef, so that's what we had when he came in for the weekend. It took forever. We had to cut our meat into tiny pieces because Mother once knew a woman who choked on a piece of roast beef and died clutching a fork in one hand and a buttered biscuit in the other.

After the dishes had been put up, we kids would pile into the big rope hammock on the porch. You could hear it groan on its hinges as the five of us scooted down to get comfortable, and whoever was on the bottom ended up with a red fanny.

In his own good time, Daddy would come out on the porch and get into the hammock with us.

At first, we would just rock slowly, listening to the sweet summer song of sea oats rustling, waves snoring and katydids fiddling away in the dunes.

"Did you ever hear the story about the Laughing Man?" he would ask.

We'd all say no, but that lie was allowed.

"Well," he'd say after a while, "I'll tell you."

And then it would start.

At first there'd be little hopscotch sounds way down in his stomach.

Then a few hiccuped chuckles.

Next, he'd wheeze and shake his shoulders, and we'd have to take a deep breath to hold it all in.

Because, you see, the whole point — the only point — of the Laughing Man's story was to see who could go the longest without joining him.

We'd stare, stern-faced and unflinching, our eyes burning in their sockets, cheek muscles squeezed so tight they hurt — while the Laughing Man went through his repertoire of laughs:

The fat-cheeked sputtering laugh, the thunder-on-the-mountain laugh, the Mortimer Snerd laugh, the howling hyenas, the mad scientist cackle . . .

Until, one by one, we exploded.

At which point, somebody started tickling somebody else, and the whole thing got so out of control the hammock turned over and dumped us all over the porch in a pile of mush.

"And that," he'd say, getting up and smoothing down his haywire hair, "is the story of the Laughing Man."

It's a silly memory, I suppose.

But I like first of all to remember him like that.

Not as the Payer of Bills, the Giver of Sermons, the Leader of the Pack.

Not the man I see in family movies, looking hardly old enough to have five children at the beach or anywhere else.

Not in the hospital with tubes in his nose and doctors pounding on his chest trying to get him so he could laugh again.

But as silly storyteller, in a hammock, at the beach.

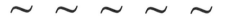

There are two kinds of people — you know them,
As you journey along life's track:
The people who take your strength from you,
And others who put it all back.
— Ralph Spaulding Cushman

SHARING OUR LOSSES

A tragic thing happened in our area
one weekend shortly before Easter
1993. The Lavies family, visiting
from Alabama, had taken the
Rainbow Falls Trail up part of Mt.
LeConte, over in the Smokies, and 13-year-old
Brad Lavies ran ahead of his parents and
somehow took a wrong turn and became
disoriented, unable to find his way back.
Search and rescue teams from the area
brought in helicopters, dogs and hundreds of
volunteers, but it was a week before they
found his body. He had fallen off a ledge and
was killed instantly. On Saturday before
Palm Sunday, about noon, they found Brad's
body, face down at the bottom of an unnamed
waterfall in a remote area of the park. This is
an open letter to his parents and to his 12-
year-old brother.

Dear Mr. and Mrs. Lavies and Chris:

We in Knoxville woke up Palm Sunday to the sad news that Brad's body had been found.

That the long and hopeful search had come to a tragic end.

Since first hearing of Brad's disappearance, this whole community has been with you.

At the checkout counter in grocery stores, at lunch booths in the heart of town, in classrooms and synagogues, in family dens and at church suppers — all week — countless people have expressed concern and compassion.

As we jogged along our quiet streets, in the early morning privacy of our own thoughts, we sent up our prayers. As we cooked supper or settled in the chair with the newspaper or shuffled the papers on our desks — a thousand vicarious pleas went up for Brad's safety.

Brad Lavies is a name we will remember.

You have no way of knowing this unless someone tells you. I took a family member to the hospital this week and sat in the waiting room while she was in surgery. As others waited for their loved ones, the conversation in every corner at some point turned to Brad and to your family's anguish.

Our son in Charleston, S.C., messaged me via computer during the week asking if Brad had been found. A neighbor, digging in the garden, waved at me on the way in from work, wanting to know if I had heard any news.

The teller at the bank was talking to her associate about how hard it must be on Brad's brother, Chris. She had children the same age as your two sons.

Everywhere I went last week people were waiting and suffering with you.

This means, of course, that your prayers and ours were answered in ways we can never fully understand.

God moves in mysterious ways, but he is certainly not so cruel as to have "caused" Brad's foot to slip or to have "willed" him to take the wrong path.

It was an accident.

God is not to blame, and neither are you.

Anyone who has ever had a 13-year-old knows how full of life they are, how eager to be independent, to do things their way. We cannot put a plastic bubble around our children. We cannot trail along beside them every step of the way. We cannot nag and holler and smother.

It's the children who are not energetic and curious who should worry us, not the ones who are. Brad was doing what kids do, and you were doing what good parents do.

What happened to your family happened, in a way, to us all because every one of us lives with these *what-ifs* in our own lives. It was a tragic turn of events that defies explaining or reason.

We point out the dangers, explain the rules, take reasonable precautions — but life is still a risk.

We can all name close calls, times when a turn of the head or an enthusiastic dash off on our own could have ended in a freak accident.

Unless we put kids on a leash, we can never control what happens: Letting them cross the street, swim in the ocean, go on their first — or fiftieth — road trip, hike a trail — it's all a risk. Deep in the heart of every parent is the fear of what might happen *if* . . .

And it happened, somehow, to Brad.

We offer to you not the insult of platitudes and easy answers, but the hope that from this unspeakable tragedy, you can draw strength from the shared grief of this community and the realization that, in some way none of us can really explain, Brad lives on in our own children, as we realize, again, because of him and what happened how precious and precarious life is.

Hopefully in the next week, as nature sings its own resurrection song, you, Brad's friends and larger family will find in it and in each other the same promise and renewal.

BAD THINGS AND GOOD PEOPLE

It was his smile that caught my eye. We hadn't been introduced, but there was a contagious friendliness about him that made me wonder if we'd met before.

When he got up to go through the buffet line, I noticed he used a cane, and by the way he moved I knew without asking it was multiple sclerosis.

His wife — they kind of looked alike, the way people do after living together for so long — helped when necessary but didn't hover.

I'd been asked by the Lions Club to speak at the banquet honoring top sixth-grade scholars from a number of area schools. It was a nice affair, but I couldn't help contrast the jiggly-wiggly, can't-sit-still energy of the honorees with the man whose nerves had become "sclerotic in many places" — which is what multiple sclerosis actually means.

My brother has multiple sclerosis. If you met him now, you wouldn't know he was once a football quarterback or a Presbyterian minister with a magic way with children or a 12th-grade heartthrob.

I'll never forget the time long ago, visiting our grandparents in North Carolina, when he took me out to the cemetery on the edge of the tobacco fields and we hopped the old Laurinburg & Southern as it crawled into town.

I once watched him eat 18 pancakes.

He taught me to burp, to drive a stick-shift car and introduced me to The Mormon Tabernacle Choir, P.D.Q. Bach, the Smothers Brothers and escargots. He covered for me when I got in past curfew and never took the steps up to his room less than two at a time.

When I went off to college, he told me if he ever caught me drinking at parties and acting crazy, he would tan my hide good.

He sang tenor in his college choir. He taught me to water-ski and to waltz and sent me postcards from his backpacking trip through France.

Now that's all gone. Except in his eyes. You can still see that part of him in his eyes: the dancing and good stories, his energy and the way he can look into your soul with a kind of scorching sincerity.

Multiple sclerosis is a progressive illness, usually striking young adults. It's more a matter of eliminating other possibilities than diagnosing it when it first begins to manifest itself.

Most often it is eyesight and balance that are first affected. My brother's early clues were double vision and a loss of equilibrium. They ruled out brain tumors, eye and heart problems. When they told us it was multiple sclerosis and that the chances were good that he could have long periods of remission, we were relieved.

But even good chances are no guarantee. Somebody has to be on the low side of the numbers.

He has double vision now and his speech is slurred, sometimes almost inaudibly. He's in a wheelchair and needs 24-hour nursing care.

The night after the Lions Club dinner, our daughter called from college. The professor had assigned the exam-paper topic for her religion course: "Why is there suffering in the world?"

"If everything that happens is God's will, then what kind of God is in control?" our daughter was asking, trying to settle in on a thesis statement. "We have to have quotes and proof and a bibliography . . . I know what I want to say. It's just that I can always think of something that argues against it . . ."

I didn't — couldn't — tell her how many times I've asked that question when I think about my brother. Why him? Why anybody? Why the man with the cane in the buffet line? And not me or you or the next-door neighbor?

Questions like that make my brother smile now. He'd be the first to let God off the hook. The silent, out-of-control growth of cells, an 18-wheeler crossing the line on a rain-slickened turn, the plug getting pulled between brain and muscles — these are not the tricks of the trade for a God of love.

"Why is there suffering" is the exam question of a Sunday morning faith in a Monday morning world.

But the answers are hard, the proof is harder and all the quotes are arguable. The best we can do is live our faith, play our hunches and — if we are lucky — find in people around us, even strangers in line at a Lions Club dinner, a light that shines through all the murky answers.

THE ENDLESS
CIRCLE OF LIFE

A week ago today, I stood in the pulpit of the Presbyterian Church in Lumberton, N.C., and bid farewell to my cousin, my best childhood friend. Presbyterian churches are not known for long eulogies, certainly not for the "testimonial" kind, but my cousin's wife had not known him as a boy, had not really known him long as a man. She asked me to talk about him, to pay tribute to him at his funeral, and I did.

Hervey — named for the uncle whose way of saying "hello" to little children was to twist their ears until they screamed for mercy — was an Eagle Scout, a graduate of Princeton and of Duke Law School, where he was a member of the Law Review. For years, he taught at Pace Law School in New York City. His health went downhill after a major heart attack a few years ago, and at his death he was awaiting a heart transplant.

He's the first of my generation to die. When that torch gets passed, it burns deep.

Hervey was an important part of my life. We came into the world two weeks apart and spent every summer of our childhood together. He was more friend than cousin — in many ways, like a brother.

I think of him when I see the Energizer commercials. When the rest of us were out of ideas, out of enthusiasm — GONE TO BED, FOR GOODNESS SAKE! — Hervey was "still going."

The commercials are right: There is nothing like an energizer.

He could make anybody laugh. He could talk you out of, or into, anything. He could outrun us all. He made us feel brave and strong, and he invented ways to have fun.

I can see him now, jumping off the garage roof and riding down on an armful of bamboo.

Forget the grammar lessons. I have never said "Hervey and I," in my whole life.

It was always me and Hervey.

Me and Hervey piled on pillows in the hammock, trying to learn to play the harmonica.

Me and Hervey sneaking into each other's rooms after we'd been "put to bed" and telling such awful ghost stories we'd tiptoe downstairs and sit on the back hall steps, close as we could get to the grown-ups talking on the porch.

Me and Hervey running across the dunes, coming to a screeching halt to see who could make the sand squeak the loudest.

Me and Hervey walking the jetties . . . putting Gaby sun oil on each other's back . . . swapping Jughead comic books . . . pushing each other off the pier . . . playing marathon games of Go Fish, Spit, Monopoly, Life — and when Hervey finished amending the rules even the people who marketed it would have been at a loss!

Those paint-by-number, sand castle summers:

Sitting for hours in other people's tied-up boats, talking about the meaning of life.

Then, suddenly summer was over.

Then, suddenly we were older.

I think about my own children now — and their cousins.

Suddenly, someday, they'll be older; suddenly, they'll realize that life is a family movie, and it's from each other we find out who we are, where we have been, where we are going.

Hervey left something of himself in everyone who knew him. He lives on in who we are and how we treat each other — and when the time comes, I'll think of him in the secret places of my heart when I, too, see the night coming.

I will miss him. My life is richer for having been his friend, his soul-sister. His death makes me sad, even angry.

I admire his spirit. He did not "go gently into that good night." He fought the good fight.

Life is not fair.

Yet I believe, as strongly as I believe anything . . . as surely as we can "know" such Amazing Grace . . . that when circumstances, or fate, or health, or when the years twist and turn and run their course, leaving us lost or spent, that you and I are given new life: happy surprises, far beyond our imagining.

The Lord gives and the Lord gathers up.

I am grateful that, in God's providence, Hervey was given to me, and I am grateful that, at last, he is at peace — and at home.

III. POLITICS, STATISTICS AND OTHER 'ICS

Probably the question I get asked the most about my job is "Where do you get your ideas?" My off-the-cuff answer is "Out of desperation" — which has more truth to it than I'd like to admit. Ask any journalist. Our "muse" is named Deadline.

Most people, I think, who write general interest columns on a regular basis would say that we just pay attention. We eavesdrop in restaurants, keep notepads beside the TV, let our minds wander in meetings, scribble stray thoughts on the back of deposit slips (then lose them), read billboards. That sort of thing.

It also helps to be an insatiable trivia hound. The information explosion and the computer age have made it cheap and painless for trivia addicts to get our fixes with incredible push-button, dial-an-anything ease.

Plus, there's always a survey or a report "just out" on anything you can think of.

And some you can't.

PLAYING THE PERCENTAGES

It reads like a nursery rhyme:
One, two, buckle my shoe; three, four,
shut the door.
Only it isn't pickup sticks Daniel Evan
Weiss is talking about in his new book.
It's the statistical ingredients of what it
means to be 100% American. It all started,
says Weiss, when he was sitting at an all-
American football game, eating an all-
American hot dog and watching the women in
heels walk by which, says Weiss, is what all-
American men do.

Suddenly he overheard an argument
between two men on what made a person a
real American. Not just birth or habits but
that certain something we all share. What
was it?

Weiss decided to find out. His "100%
American" is an inch-thick book of polls,
reports and indexes of what Americans do,

think, wear, believe and are.

It is, I suppose, the closest thing to a recipe for American Pie we'll ever come upon. There are 288 "ingredients" — that is, statistical findings — gleaned from the bean counters of a variety of private, business and government agencies.

Here is a buckle-my-shoe sampling, FYI:

1% of Americans read the Bible more than once a day.

2% of American wives who use devices for sexual stimulation during lovemaking use feathers.

3% of Americans think Elvis Presley was history's most exciting figure.

4% of American cheese is Swiss cheese.

5% of American high school seniors drink every day.

6% of Americans walk to work.

7% of Americans think God is more like a mother than a father figure.

8% of Americans receive food stamps.

9% of Americans often have deja vu.

10% of American babies are unwanted at the time of conception.

15% of American 17-year-olds believe the Spanish knight who attacked windmills thinking they were giants was Zorro.

20% of Americans under 18 live in poverty.

25% of Americans think their presence at a sporting event will influence its outcome.

30% of American teenage girls feel homosexuality is an acceptable alternative life-style.

35% of American college men say they might commit a rape if there were no chance of getting caught.

40% of American wives 40 years old and older have had an extramarital affair.

45% of American women wear uncomfortable shoes because they think they look good.

50% of Americans do not read books.

55% of Americans have little or no interest in hosting the Johnny Carson show.

60% of American women think motherhood is the best thing about being a woman.

65% of Americans like baked beans.

70% of Americans own running shoes but don't run.

75% of American women wear the wrong size bra.

80% of Americans do not discuss fees up front with their doctors.

85% of Americans would remarry their spouse if they had it to do over again.

90% of American refrigerators are white or almond.

91% of American airline passengers are discount fares.

92% of American women use deodorant.

93% of Americans think it is very important for parents to spend more time with children.

94% of American men would change something about their looks if they could.

95% of Americans believe in God.

96% of American parents of children under 18 say their children have never had problems with the law.

97% of American grocery stores offer paper bags.

98% of American households have at least one television.

99% of American kindergarten teachers are female.

The only thing I can think of right off the bat that is 100% American is Mark Twain. What did he have to say about the numbers game?

"There are three kinds of lies — lies, damned lies and statistics."

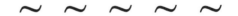

Forty-eight percent of your friends peek in your medicine cabinet when they use the bathroom at your house.

Barry Sinrod and Mel Poretz's book, "Do You Do It With The Lights On?" gets the scoop on those little deep-dark secrets . . . like, for instance:

• How many people have walked into the wrong rest room by accident? Sixty percent.

• How many people have had sex with a third person in the room? Thirty-four percent.

• How many people have made love at the office? Thirty percent.

A PAINT-BY-NUMBER POLL

Had Norman Rockwell been in the Sequoyah Elementary School gym on Election Day, he would have been one busy painter.

It would have taken all his burnt oranges and early November magentas just to get up the walkway, then a whole palette of red, white and blue to capture the living canvas inside.

This country was founded by Presbyterians — and even the ones that weren't sure acted like they were. Presbyterians do everything (to quote from the handbook) "decently and in order."

Thank goodness.

How else could you get what I'd guess were 300 people standing shoulder-to-shoulder in a hot gym, waiting up to two hours to cast their votes?

A few people anticipated the long lines

and brought something to read: Cormac McCarthy's new book. A
computer manual. A collection of Canadian poetry. The morning
newspaper.

One kid in a leftover Halloween dalmatian costume made
shadow puppets in the luscious sunlight spilling through the
windows and out on the floor like ghost lemonade.

A father, trying to explain the democratic process to his
toddler (who had better things to do than stare at people's knees),
finally gave up.

"Why don't you just tell the lady by the curtain who you want
so we can go home?" the youngster asked. Great idea.

"We'll talk about it later," said Dad.

The conversation around me was pure over-the-fence
Americana:

Susie Somebody's gall bladder.

Madonna's book. Have you seen it? Oh, my goodness, no.

Finding a place to park.

Let's do lunch.

Wasn't it awful about so-and-so's marriage?

If you put a water heater in the attic, you'd better set it in a
flash pan, just in case.

. . . a running commentary on life in the suburbs.

Nobody I heard was talking politics.

It got testy after a while, standing decently in the stale air,
with its faint smell of kids coming in from kickball.

Still everyone followed, the way grown-ups are supposed to,
the GYM RULES posted in large teacher-print on the cinder block
wall:

Walk quietly and stay in line.
Listen and follow directions.
Ignore inappropriate behavior.
Do not touch anyone.

There were a few slipups, especially when it came to that last
one. Two neighbors hugged each other. One little boy kept
punching his father, trying to get his attention so he could ask
about the TEN FEET warning taped to the floor in front of the
voting booth.

"Don't they mean *toes*, Dad? . . . Dad? . . . Why do they say
TEN FEET, Dad. Nobody has TEN FEET . . . Dad?'

And — just as I was thinking how much Norman Rockwell would have loved the huge American flag made from construction paper handprints and tacked up on the stage curtain to welcome us — my husband came up from behind and broke the _no touching_ rule AND the _ignore inappropriate behavior_ rule.

Tapping me on the shoulder, he whispered into my ear: "Spit out the chewing gum."

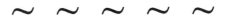

"We are the only people in the world required by law to take large amounts of money from strangers and then act as if it has no effect on our behavior." — Rep. Barney Frank, D-Mass., on campaign fund-raising.

FIRST LADY FASHIONS

Hillary-watching is in full fashion now. We can even get all the First Lady scoop in a new magazine called The Hillary Clinton Quarterly.

She's already upset the apple cart in the clothes world by saying she plans to continue shopping in department stores like regular people.

Frank Marfiote, publisher of The Hillary Clinton Quarterly, is busy second-guessing what retailers should stock up on, following our new first lady's suit.

And so far, says Marfiote, those suits are mostly knits, bright colors and worn with a scarf.

Whenever I get down in the dumps, I can always thank my lucky stars I don't have to spend my days writing about how Hillary Clinton styles her hair. My idea of great investigative journalism is not trying to read labels off her blouses.

Anyway, Marfiote thinks we should look for a rebirth of scarves and headbands.

Uh oh.

Headbands give me headaches and scarves seem to come alive the minute they get around my neck. I have been known to stand up in the middle of church and rip one off before it choked me to death.

Nevertheless, despite fashion dropouts like me, the big news, for some people at least, is that Hillary Clinton's legacy to the fashion world is to be the scarf and headband look.

(Do you reckon we'll ever get a first lady who wears hospital scrubs and sleeps in her husband's socks?)

Every modern first lady has made a different fashion statement.

Jackie Kennedy's was the pillbox hat.

Now, I hesitate to mention this because anybody who knows me will surely think I am making this up — but I actually made a pillbox hat for myself during the Kennedy era. At the time, I was in my domestic incarnation and signed up for a sewing course at the local YWCA. For months I worked on my outfit: a blue tweed suit, matching shoes and pillbox hat.

When I finally finished, I put it all on to model for my husband who looked up from the newspaper and said, in a nice pastorly way, "Oh, my goodness, what have you got on yourself? You look like a cross between the Queen Mother and Tinkerbell. Is it Halloween?"

Or words to that effect.

Rosalynn Carter was more my speed, with her shirtwaist dresses. She wore clothes you could actually do things in. Like walk and talk and stir up a salad. Of course, lots of people were disappointed in Rosalynn's manner of dress. Not fancy enough, they said. I once heard a group of women say she brought dishonor to the presidency because she fired all the designers and dressed like a bag lady.

Which hurt my feelings because she's the only first lady who ever looked like she would feel at home in my closet.

Nancy Reagan? The basic red dress.

In negative sizes and laundered in industrial-strength starch.

Barbara Bush was a godsend to those of us for whom "fine jewelry" means a painted macaroni pin made at day camp or a gold-filled circle pin your mother told you never to be without in case she got hit by a truck and you had to go to a funeral.

You'll thank me for telling you all this Hillary Clinton news in time for you to add headbands and scarves to your shopping list. I'm sure you already have a Reagan-red dress in upgraded sizes, faux Bush pearls and probably at least one Carter-ite shirtwaist somewhere in the back of your closet.

If you don't have a pillbox hat, never mind. Only organ-grinders' monkeys wear them these days.

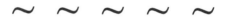

There's a lake in Massachusetts that the Indians called Chargoggagoggmanchaug-gagoggchaubagungamaugg — which translates into "neutral fishing spot."

Those Indians sound like some of our politicians: takes them a long time to say something simple.

OUR DAYS ARE NUMBERED

Like sand through the hourglass . . . so are the days of our lives."
Those words make me think of folding diapers.

Back in that other lifetime when I had two children in (cloth) diapers, every afternoon during their naps, I used to unload the dryer and park myself in front of "my" soap opera.

Those sudsy words swooped me off into a world where life was a nail-biting series of disasters, scandals and freak accidents. In one story line, a man got amnesia and fell in love with his own sister who had been away in a convent since she was a teenager and didn't recognize him when they — ta dum! — accidentally ran into each other in New York City after she decided to leave the sisterhood to become a brain surgeon . . .

The days of my life were real snoozers

compared to what went on in the Horton family.

I haven't watched "Days of Our Lives" in twenty years, but the sand is still flowing through the hourglass every afternoon at 2. Macdonald Carey (father of those star-crossed lovers) still starts the show by reminding us that, like sand, our days are numbered.

Marc McCutcheon, a science writer for OMNI and Science Digest, says there's a way we can actually count those sands, based on medical research and good-guess probabilities. In "The Compass in Your Nose," he devotes a whole chapter to "The Days of Our Lives" — the emphasis here being on life span rather than amnesia and nuns.

His "life-expectancy quiz" is typical of questionnaires now used by insurance companies and health-care agencies. There is an obvious margin of error here — but, warns McCutcheon, don't take it too lightly:

"Odds are that your predicted life span will be quite close."

Here's how to figure it.

Start with the number 74.

If you are male, subtract 2; female, add 4.

If you live in a city with over 2 million people, subtract 2. If you live in a rural area with a population under 10,000, add 2.

If any grandparent lived to be 85, add 2; if all four grandparents lived to be 80, add 6; if either parent died of a stroke or heart attack before the age of 50, subtract 4.

If any immediate relative under 50 has ever had cancer or a heart condition or diabetes since childhood, subtract 3.

If you earn over $50,000 a year, subtract 2.

If you finished college, add 1. If you have a graduate or professional degree, add 2 more.

If you live with a spouse or a friend, add 5. Subtract 1 for every 10 years you've lived alone since age 25.

If you work behind a desk, subtract 3.

If your work is physically demanding, add 3.

If you exercise 3 to 5 times a week for at least 30 minutes, add 4; if twice a week, add 2. If you sleep more than 10 hours per night, subtract 4.

If you are aggressive, tense or easily angered, subtract 3; generally relaxed and easygoing, add 3.

If you are happy most of the time, add 1.

If you are unhappy most of the time, subtract 2.

If you smoke half a pack a day, subtract 3; a pack, subtract 7; 2 packs or more, subtract 8.

If you drink more that 1 1/2 ounces of liquor a day, subtract 1.

If overweight 10-30 pounds, subtract 2; 30-50 pounds, subtract 4; 50 or more pounds, subtract 8.

If you have an annual physical exam, add 2.

If you are 30-40 years old, add 2; 40-50, add 3; 50-70, add 4; over 70, add 5.

That's the number of sands in your hourglass.

You get a "plus" next to that number if your blood pressure is less than 130/75, your cholesterol less than 200 and resting pulse rate less than 60 beats a minute. Also add a plus if you are a light eater, don't skip breakfast and presently have a pet.

Give yourself a "minus" if you are easily winded or have no social contacts besides spouse.

Counting sands in an hourglass is, at best, an exercise in frustration. But at least it makes us see that time is slipping by.

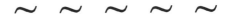

"Old" is always — as far as I'm concerned — anybody who has had about 20 more birthdays than I have. An article in "Special Report" says I'm wrong.

According to a recent poll conducted by Omnitel, here's the scoop.

When is a woman old? Women say at 69, men say at 59.

When is a man old? Women say 70, men say at 65.

. . . and you know what the Bible says in Ecclesiastes:

"As the clear light is upon a holy candlestick, so is the beauty of a face in ripe age."

Which, of course, is true. That's why we often dine by candlelight at our house.

FRUIT PUNCH

There's a new theory out about fat — or rather, fat people. It goes something like this: Every baby comes into this world with one of two words written on its DNA. "Pear" or "Apple."

Whichever the case may be, it's a harmless word, just sitting there minding its own business, not bothering anybody and making no difference whatsoever to anything — unless a person starts overeating and not exercising. Then it's only a matter of time before that word starts directing traffic, telling all the blobs of fat exactly where to go.

That's why, say researchers, overweight people are one of two shapes: round like an apple or blossom-hipped like a pear.

It depends on what shape you start out with as to what you'll get when blown up.

Kind of like a balloon.

Doctors are now saying that apple-shaped people are more prone to diseases than pear-shaped people.

Here's how to find out which orchard you belong in:

(1) Measure your waist at its smallest point without sucking in your gut. (2) Find the place on your hips that is the largest and measure it without pulling on the tape. (3) Divide waist measurement by hip measurement. If the ratio is above 0.80 for women and 0.95 for men, you are an apple and, so say the medical gurus, at a higher risk for "several diseases" than your pear peers.

Of course, you really don't need a tape measure or a mind for math to know whether you are a Golden Delicious or a Bartlett.

You don't even need a doctor.

Just look in the mirror.

If the mirror asks, "When's it due?" — you're an apple.

If it says, "Where's the partridge?" — you're a pear.

Or try to buy some clothes. If you need a size, say, 8 at the top and an 18 at the bottom, you're a pear. Apples wear 8s at the top and bottom, 18s in the middle.

But the fact of the matter is apples and pears aren't the only two shapes to figure.

There are a lot of other fruits in the loom.

What about bananas? A bunch of people are banana-shaped: same size all the way down, tall and slightly bent. James Stewart, for one. Strom Thurmond, for another.

The alien who visits agent Cooper in "Twin Peaks" is a perfect banana.

Then there are the watermelons like Roseanne Barr, although some of you may argue she is more of a strawberry or even a persimmon. Dom DeLuise and Pavarotti are better examples.

George Burns is a raisin, Mickey Rooney is a pumpkin, and Dolly Parton is more grapefruit than grape, apple or pear. Or possibly a honeydew.

Tim Conner is a perfect jujube.

Billy Joel is a fuzzy peach.

Charlie Chaplin was a plum. Pee Wee Herman is a kumquat, Jesse Helms an onion, and Marilyn Monroe was what you'd get if you crossed passion fruit with a cherry tomato.

Add a little hagberry to that recipe, and you come up with Madonna.

Of course, some people aren't fruits at all. They are vegetables. Queen Victoria was an eggplant. Lily Tomlin is a bean. Joan Rivers is either broccoli or leeks — I can't decide which. Molly Ringwald is a perfect carrot. Bart's mom, Marge Simpson, is a blue horseradish.

Ted Koppel is celery with wilted leaves.

Sam Nunn is a turnip.

Nancy Reagan is an asparagus.

Jonathan Winters is pure corn.

Then there are the nuts.

Whether you are a fruit or a vegetable, you have to be a little off your rocker to get into this sort of thing, but go ahead. Get crazy. I bet if you put your mind to it, you can think of a whole bunch of produce pals.

My husband doesn't go in for silly parlor games like this at all, but he thought of one right off.

He said I was a fruitcake.

THE FIRST SHALL
BE LAST, SOMETIMES

W e are No. 1 . . . and we're going to stay that way!" President Bush made this battle cry the prayer and passion of his administration and wobbly campaign.

Of course, being No. 1 is not always a good thing. Anybody knows that. A new book that uses this cheer as its title — "We're Number One," by Andrew L. Shapiro — proves this point very well.

Using data from the Organization for Economic Cooperation and Development, United Nations, the World Values Survey, the World Health Organization and other international agencies, Shapiro charts where America stands and falls in the New World Order.

It's a roller coaster ride through inconsistencies, ironies and contradictions.

The American Dream — slash — Nightmare.

We're No. 1 in big homes, and we're No. 1 in homelessness.

We're No. 1 in highest-paid athletes and last in teacher salaries.

We're No. 1 in percentage of young people who say premarital sex should be avoided, and we're No. 1 in teenage pregnancies.

We're No. 1 in time spent watching television and last of all in book titles published per capita.

Throughout the book, Shapiro compares us with 18 major industrial nations, those countries that are most comparable to the United States in social and economic development: Australia, Austria, Belgium, Canada, Denmark, Finland, France, Germany, Ireland, Italy, Japan, the Netherlands, New Zealand, Norway, Spain, Sweden, Switzerland, and the United Kingdom.

The first issue the book tackles is health and medical care. Shapiro names this chapter "Chronic Disorder."

Our per capita spending on health care is the highest of any nation in the world, yet we are the only Western democracy without a national health-care plan covering all citizens. Two-thirds of those Americans polled were in favor of a more equitable, nationalized health-care system like Canada's.

In a chapter he calls "Pieties and Priorities," Shapiro maps out what we say we believe and what we actually do.

It's frightening.

We are No. 1 in getting married, No. 1 in still believing in the sanctity of marriage . . . yet No. 1 in divorce and No. 1 in single parent families.

We're No. 1 in private spending on education and No. 17 in public spending on education.

No. 9 in early childhood education. No. 15 in days spent in school each year.

No. 1 in percentage of students who *say* they're good at math, but last place in percentage of students who actually are good at math.

We're No. 1 in garbage per capita, yet No. 14 in recycling paper, No. 16 in recycling glass.

Probably the strangest and perhaps the most easily "fixed" contradiction is our schizophrenia in the area of voting rights and actions. We are No. 1 in percentage of population that says they take an active interest in politics but last place in voter turnout.

Half of America never shows up at the polls. The number of Americans who say they vote is about 13 million more than actually do.

Part of the reason is that we make it so complicated. Political analyst G. Bingham Powell calls our registration system "truly Byzantine." Residency requirements, with more than half of us moving at least once every five years, make it difficult for many to vote.

Or too complicated to bother.

In Australia and New Zealand, voting is a law and those who do not are fined.

At any rate, Shapiro's book is not good bedtime reading, but it is convincing evidence that there are a number of areas where America needs to wake up.

~ ~ ~ ~ ~

Two firsts in American history happened on Aug. 9 in 1974. Richard M. Nixon became the first person to resign the presidency. His intention was announced on TV the night before, but the papers were signed Aug. 9.

That same day, Gerald R. (Quick! What does the "R" stand for?) Ford became the first person to serve as vice president and president without being elected to either office. (The "R" stands for Rudolph.)

Nixon is maybe the most-quoted and quoted-about modern president in who-said-what anthologies. My personal favorite Nixonism is "If I had to live my life over, I would have liked to have ended up as a sportswriter."

Runner-up: "People said my language was bad, but, Jesus, you should have heard LBJ!"

I reckon He did.

BURNING BRA-VOS!

Over and over women heard in voices of tradition and Freudian sophistication that they could desire no greater destiny than to glory in their own femininity (and) to pity the neurotic, unfeminine, unhappy women who wanted to be poets or physicians or presidents."

It reads like a piece of absurd ancient history, but in 1963 these words went off like a bomb in kitchens and car pools around the country. They come from the first chapter of Betty Friedan's book, "The Feminine Mystique."

In 1963, Friedan, a suburban housewife, looked up from the sink, so to speak, and asked a question.

"Is this all there is?"

A good question, but a dangerous one, especially when referring to the scrub-a-dub

103

chores of housewifedom, or the image women saw of themselves in TV commercials, or the intellectual frustrations of having more brain than it takes to read the backs of cereal boxes and "Good Night Moon" for the 100th time.

Friedan answered her own question and, before the ink was dry, her answer became a best-seller, reprinted, excerpted, quoted and translated into more than 15 languages.

It took issue with the roles women had been assigned — handed down like antique chairs too old for anybody to sit in, or holy writ nobody understood but wouldn't dare question.

In 1968, three years after the publication of "The Feminine Mystique," Gloria Steinem — whose grandmother was president of the Ohio Women's Suffrage Association back in 1908 — needed to gather some information for her political column in New York magazine. She began looking into how women were being treated in the work force, in politics, in history textbooks. Already an established and articulate writer, she quickly became a well-known advocate for equal rights.

Friedan and Steinem made people think, and they made people mad.

"American children suffer too much mother and too little father," said Steinem. She called housework names Mr. Clean never thought of.

Friedan's statements started everything from classroom debates to family feuds: "American women no longer know who they are." . . . "It is easier to live through someone else than to become complete yourself."

With time, Friedan started the National Organization for Women, Steinem started Ms. magazine, and the two together started "the women's movement."

A misnomer, to be sure. Women have always been on the move, but mostly in the background. Mostly in support roles. Some even behind veils. Why was it that when men went into the "library" to talk of important things, women were expected to powder their noses or go back to their knitting? Or take up tennis and shopping?

For most women, it was love or hate at first sight when they read or heard what Friedan and Steinem had to say.

"Yes!" said some. "Hogwash!" said others.

Even Redbook got a surprise. In an Are-You-Fulfilled? survey, women blew the charts with repressed frustration. An article in the first issue of Ms. magazine titled "I Want A Wife" had suburban, middleclass housewives gasping for air after laughing themselves sick. It's a classic. If you missed it, do yourself a favor and dig up a copy at the library.

We aren't out of the woods by a long shot, but we have come a long way. At least far enough to have Women's History Month marked on the calendar. But then, lots of things have their own month: pickles, fire safety, kidneys and prune breakfasts. Just to name a few.

Whether or not you agreed with Friedan and Steinem — and they were very controversial — women owe them a round of applause for encouraging women to think about what we are doing, to choose carefully and from conviction the work we do, and not to treat life as a spectator sport.

Friedan and Steinem sent Phyllis Schlafly into a frenzy and sent political platform writers back to the drawing board. They had mothers and daughters giving each other what we call in our house "the hairy eyeball" . . . that frowning, disapproving look that says, "I can't believe what just came out of your mouth!"

But read again those words from "The Feminine Mystique," and the fact that they seem hardly up for debate at all — whether you are Mother Hubbard or a brain surgeon — explains why these two women have a significant place in history.

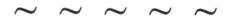

According to a study at the University of Michigan, a woman who "marries up" to a man better educated than she tends to live longer than one whose mate is her equal in education.

GET OFF THE POT

Just when you think you've heard everything, you hear something else. Hot off the wires, as they say, comes a comment made by one of our distinguished state senators that makes you wonder if they haven't found the missing link after all, right there in Nashville.

It's Neanderthal reasoning at its best.

Or worst, depending on how you feel about potty parity.

Potty parity?

It's the newest word (although it's hard to tell, they are coined so quickly) in equality politics and, taken to its lowest common denominator, means "how come it takes women so long to go to the bathroom, and so what if it does?"

Before you close this book and go off in a huff, saying such things shouldn't be discussed in print, let me assure you that's exactly what they are discussing in Nashville:

How many ladies' rooms should there be in public buildings? More than men's rooms? The same number?

Ask any woman — from Donna Reed to Sinead O'Connor — who has ever tried to freshen up in a busy airport between planes, and you have your answer. Especially if she's traveling with a man.

He could grow a beard waiting for her.

Or check the lines outside the ladies' room at, say, intermissions — even, or maybe I should say especially, at high class events like operas and symphonies. The men wander in and out of their room in time to visit the refreshment stand and chat with their buddies. But the mezzanine lights flicker long before the toilets finish flushing in the ladies' room. In fact, if you want to get a seat at all, pardon the pun, you better run while folks are still clapping.

Why does it take so long for women?

Try it sometime, all ye who don't know from experience.

Put on underwear, pantyhose, slip, skirt, blouse, coat, scarf, pocketbook and maybe a small child or two tucked under your arms. Now go inside a cubicle the size of a phone booth (if you are lucky; try these gymnastics in a gas station that is cutting corners and you're liable to break something). Now, find a place to put your pocketbook, check the paper situation, pull everything down and when the time comes, pull it all back up where it belongs.

Don't fuss at me for being so basic here. This arrangement was not my idea. In fact, I remember standing in line, standing in line, standing in line, standing in line — first on one foot and then another — at the movie theater when a woman next to me whispered, "God is a man!"

So, what's this about potty parity?

The bill before the state legislature would require all public buildings in the future to increase the number of rest rooms for women.

Sen. John Ford, D-Memphis, who opposes the legislation, has another solution. He's the Neanderthal up there in the opening paragraph. He says forget adding more ladies' rooms. We women should just drink less.

Yes, you heard me right. He says women should drink less because it takes them longer to go to the bathroom.

"Women," he said during committee discussions of the so-called potty parity bill, "ought not to drink so much beer, or water, or Pepsi, or whatever it is."

Why not make women wear diapers? Or catheters?

Maybe we could have His and Hers drinking fountains and make the cups smaller on Hers.

The bill, by the way, passed the Senate General Welfare Committee and will next be considered by the full Senate.

Frankly, I don't have a lot of emotion invested in this issue, but I hope John what's-his-name (toilets even have a man's name!) was kidding and doesn't face the big issues with such laughable logic.

The whole thing reminds me of the joke about the Sunday school teacher who asked the class if anyone knew where God lives.

"In my parents' bathroom!" says one little boy.

"The bathroom???" teacher says, stalling for time to handle this one.

"Yeah. Every morning, my dad stands outside the bathroom, beating on the door and yelling, 'Good Lord, are you still in there?'"

IV. FAMILY AND OTHER FRUSTRATIONS

It's like the day our daughter came home from preschool and asked how come everybody in our family had married one of our relatives: "You married Dad. Gran married Granddaddy. Uncle Bobby married Aunt Becky . . . is that normal?"

Ah, yes. Very. We go through this life hooked onto each other like boxcars behind the Little Engine That Could. Over the bridges, up the hills, through the tunnels. Sometimes pushing, sometimes pulling each other. Only together do we make it.

ECHOES OF
THE FUTURE

There's a familiar giggle coming from behind a Fruit Loops cereal box. A fan wheezes in the corner of the kitchen, losing its battle against the heat. The giggling stops, starts again.

Then, bare feet hit the floor and a screen door slams.

Such is the music of all my summers. Since before I can remember, our family has come in loaded-down station wagons to join aunts and cousins at Wrightsville Beach. We brought our children to the same cottages that my parents brought the five of us to back when cars were not allowed on the island and everyone rode the streetcar over the bridge from the mainland.

Our son George had a special name for the sound of our tires as they hit the drawbridge over the Inland Waterway.

"Trip noise," he called it. It was the sweet sound of summer.

Other sounds echo down the years every time my mind makes those trips back in time: The slap and pop of towels hung out to dry on the upstairs porch, dancing in the wind like a row of pastel paper dolls. The drumrolls of a midnight thunderstorm. The giggles.

This year the giggles come from a new person in our family. My grandniece. My mama's first great-grandchild.

In time, there will be others, but for now she's the star of the show. Like her daddy was that first summer he came to Wrightsville with his mother, my oldest sister. He was just-born, the newest baby I'd ever seen up close. He was so little, I didn't see how all those tiny parts could work. I worried something might go wrong, and the fans would hide the sounds of distress coming from his crib. Sometimes I just sat and watched him breathe.

By the next year, he had a sister — and a cousin. Before the stork had finished its rounds, my mother had 15 grandchildren, each brought, come summertime, to Wrightsville for whatever rite of passage the summer required.

For a 2-year-old, it might be a trip down the water slide. For a 5-year-old, his first summer of catching sand fiddlers and putting them down other people's bathing suits.

For a 12-year-old, pulling Spanish mackerel in two at a time on an all-day fishing trip.

For teenagers, the first tag-along adventure with older cousins to a beer joint, or a first kiss under the boardwalk, trying not to let on they were nervous, uncomfortable and would really rather be back at the cottage playing Monopoly.

The hammocks drug bottom, piled high with our children, the way they had with the five of us before time started going in fast forward.

Our children sat on the same creaky porch rail and spit watermelon seeds into the dunes; played Pokeno on the same gritty gameboard we had and walked to the pier to buy fireballs like we had done a hundred times before them, back when our taste buds were young and our back teeth unfilled.

Time has a way of interrupting traditions, especially when children grow older. This summer is the first summer since our first child was born that we have not gone as a family to

Wrightsville. One daughter is working in New Mexico. Another is in California. Our son is in school in South Carolina. No longer do we plan their summers and, until school and jobs are settled, neither do they.

So we went without them, taking the new interstate that makes such a beeline we never even had to slow down for a traffic light — making those long, hot trips on the two-lane roads of my childhood seem like trips through a foreign country now swallowed up in time.

My mother was there and my older sister's family. Both her children are married now. They have always blazed the trail of "firsts."

And there behind the Fruit Loops, giggling that giggle that echoes around the room and down the years, is the first of the next generation. She'll be the one to take my grandchildren someday on their first unchaperoned walk to the pier for bubble gum. Or out on the Sunfish. Or up in the lifeguard stand after supper for a bowl of boiled peanuts and a ghost story.

And if all the rules are followed, someday my daughter's child will look into the crib of her child and see the future.

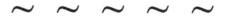

For reasons yet unclear to scientists, most women carry babies in their left arms. Eighty percent of all chimps, gorillas and orangutans also cradle their babies in their left arms.

The latest theory is that since the left side of the body sends information to the right side of the brain, and the right side of the brain deals with emotions — then if you hold a baby on your left, you can better pick up on the baby's emotional signals. Right?

Personally, I think it's so mom can have her best arm free to do all the things she has to do while holding her baby. Ever tried to tie a shoe with one left hand?

TALKING MACHINES

Hello. You have reached the Hughs residence. We can't come to the phone right now, but if you leave your name and number at the sound of the tone, we'll get back with you as soon as we can.

"Mom, this is Claire. I have these awful pains in my stomach, and I almost fainted in chemistry class. Call me when you come in. 'Bye."

Hi there! Boy, do you have THE RIGHT NUMBER! This is Claire and Meredith's room. We're out having a wild and crazy time with rich fraternity guys. Unless you are our parents. If you are our parents, we are both in the library working on our Phi Beta Kappa research project. But, whoever you are, near or far . . . oooh wee ohhh wah wah . . . when you hear the tone, rap in the phone . . . doo dee dah dah doo dee dah.

"Claire, this is Mom. I thought you were sick! I don't like that phone message. It's . . . well . . . besides, it's too long. I'm glad you are well enough to go out. If you feel bad tomorrow, go to the infirmary."

Hello. You have reached the Hughs residence. We can't come to the phone right now, but if you leave your name and number at the sound of the tone, we'll get back with you as soon as we can.

"Hey, Mom and Dad. This is George. Guess what? Friday classes were canceled, and I got someone to work for me this weekend, so I'm coming home. See you in a couple of hours. I'm bringing four friends. Wait! I forgot. There'll be five. Six, counting me. Don't go to any trouble."

Hello. You have reached the Hughs residence. We can't come to the phone right now, but if you leave your name and number at the sound of the tone, we'll get back with you as soon as we can.

"Mom, it's me again. I feel awful, but I can't go to the infirmary. They don't know anything. I got these green-looking pills from a girl down the hall whose uncle is a doctor and gave them to her when she had mono, but we're not sure how many to take. Everybody says they're positive it's mono. I definitely have fever. Meredith said she'd never felt such a hot forehead, and I'm sooooooo tired. Call as soon as you come in. I'm going to bed. Oh, we changed the message. 'Bye."

Hello. If you have a message for Claire or Meredith, leave it at the sound of the tone.

"Claire? CLAIRE. Claire, wake up! Hello? HELLO. IS ANYBODY THERE? THERE MAY BE A SICK SLEEPING CHILD WITH ADVANCED MONO WHO IS IN A COMA AND NEEDS HER MOTHER!!!"

Hello. You have reached the Hughs residence. We can't come to the phone right now, but if you leave your name and number at the sound of the tone, we'll get back with you as soon as we can.

"Dad, this is McNair. Uh. Hmmmm. Does the car insurance cover cracks in the windshield? . . . Like from pebbles that get thrown up and hit the window? It's kind of a big crack. Maybe it was more like a rock. I mean, it's not that big. I've got a piece of cardboard over it, but it's raining. Um. Well, never mind. Don't worry. 'Bye."

Hello. You have reached the Hughs residence. We can't come to the phone right now, but if you leave your name and number at the sound of the tone, we'll get back with you as soon as we can.

"Mom? I got your message. It was embarrassing. Don't scream in the phone like that. I think I was just tired. I feel better now. Don't bother calling back. This is beach weekend. Oh, could you send me McNair's black short strapless for the prom? I need it tomorrow night. Thanks. 'Bye."

Hello. You have reached the Hughs residence. We can't come to the phone right now, but if you leave your name and number at the sound of the tone, we'll get back with you as soon as we can.

"Mom. This is George. I forgot my house key. We're at . . . HEY, WHAT'S THE NAME OF THIS PLACE? . . . Exit 360 Quick 'n Go . . . something like that. Call us . . . well, no. We'll just call back. 'Bye. Wait! I almost forgot. There are eight of us. 'Bye."

Hello. You have reached the Hughs residence. We have bashed our answering machine with an ax. We don't want any more messages. So, when you hear the sound of the tone, hang up and call someone else. 'Bye.

DRIVEN TO DISTRACTION

E ver played "20 Questions" with a 4-year-old?

Pick one. It can be your own, a niece or nephew, a grandchild, a neighbor. Four-year-olds are not shy if you give them half a chance. Put him or her in the front seat of the car next to you, turn off the radio, and start driving.

First one question, then another. And another. And another. And another. And another. It goes something like this:

How much does a tree weigh?

I don't know.

What does it feel like to be a worm?

I don't know.

Did you ask a lot of questions when you were little?

Yes.

Then how come you don't know anything?

I'll try harder. Ask me something else.

Are all skies blue?
Yes.
How do you know? Have you seen them all? Maybe way over yonder the sky is green and the grass is blue. Maybe, huh?
It's all one sky. It's all hooked together. God probably thought about other colors, but I think he ended up with the right choice, don't you?
Nope. I would have colored the sky GREEN and the grass PURPLE. Do you think God might ever change his mind? Huh? Are you listening?
I'm thinking, I'm thinking. Sometimes God does change the colors of the sky. Have you ever seen him do that?
You mean like sunsets? Once when we left the tent up in the backyard, the grass under it turned brown.
It's nice of God to make colors change, don't you think?
Yeah, but it sure made my daddy mad about the grass.
Do you like to ride in the car?
Yeah. What makes the car drive?
Well . . .
Is it fun to drive?
Well . . .
What is the hardest thing about driving?
Well . . .
Do you get tired of driving?
Well . . .
Can I drive?
No.
Riding in the car for a long time makes my weer hurt.
Your what?
Weer. You know. The back part of your lap.
Driving makes my rrr-ear hurt.
Mine too.
No, I mean it's "rrr" instead of "www." Want some gum? Here's a big piece. Chew that for a while.
Wham ard reersh madove?
Don't try to talk and chew at the same time.
What are rears made of?
Same thing as shoulders and arms.
What are shoulders and arms made of?

Calcium and marrow.

What is calcium and marrow made of?

Uh, metallic components and blood, I think.

What's blood ma . . .

Hey! I got an idea. Why don't you tell me some answers and I will try to come up with the right question. Ever played that before?

You mean like "Jeopardy?"

Sure. Like "Jeopardy."

OK. The . . . answer . . . is . . . ummmmm . . . A HUNDRED TWO ZILLION KABILLION.

Is that how tall the sky is?

Nope.

How many stars there are?

Nope.

I give up.

It's how old you are. Ha ha ha ha ha Ha ha ha Ha ha ha ha ha ha Ha ha ha Ha ha ha ha ha ha . . .

~ ~ ~ ~ ~

Raindrops on roses and whiskers on kittens didn't score big with a group of kids tested by Sesame Street Magazine. Asked to name their favorite things, some 23,030 little readers chose Barbie dolls, Teenage Mutant Ninja Turtles, pizza and spaghetti. "Twinkle Twinkle Little Star" heads the favorite song list; blue and pink are favorite colors. And they like cats better than dogs. Vegetables are the third favorite food and "Jesus Loves Me" is at the top of the charts.

SLEEP IN HEAVENLY PEACE

N ow I lay me down to sleep . . . "
How many of us put ourselves to bed
with those words we learned back
when life seemed simple and
prayers were memorized?

I used to worry about the next part: "If I
should die before I wake, I pray thee, Lord,
my soul to take." But those were the first
words that came to my mind as we stood over
my mother-in-law's bed and watched her
sleep for the last time. For her, the words had
come true.

At 6, they'd seemed morbid.

At 86, it was a blessing.

We'd brought her to live with us last
summer because of failing health. She knew
and we knew that time was running out. She
died in her sleep early one morning. We took
her back to southwest Georgia for the
funeral, and she is buried next to her

husband of over 50 years.

We in the family joked that it must have been quite a reunion in heaven that Wednesday morning when she stole quietly away to join him.

"Hi, monkey," she would say.

"Hi, bud," he'd reply.

Nobody knows how those nicknames got started. I'm not even sure they knew, really. Her candle burned low after he died two years ago. They had been friends since they were 7 years old, and there was almost no memory or important thing in her life that could be separated from him.

Together they raised two sons and two grandsons. She nursed her mother-in-law, an uncle and a cousin through long illnesses. Then, for some eight years, she stayed beside her husband's bed, making sure the hose from the oxygen tank was not rubbing against his neck, fixing him ham sandwiches just the way he liked them and refusing to leave his side for any reason except to sit in the living room when the grandchildren came to visit. After he died, her heart lost its energy, but she never could get used to having things done for her, and she never spoke in the first person. It was always "we" — even when lying in a hospital bed in a single room.

She was a Scout leader and Sunday school teacher to half the grown folks that side of town. No telling how many cupcakes she'd baked for classroom parties or how many casseroles she'd taken to sick folks. When I first met her, she couldn't pull in a filling station or stop off at the drugstore without calling a dozen people by their first names.

So, it was fitting — and deeply moving — that as we rode behind the hearse to the cemetery that Saturday morning, traffic came to a halt to let the procession by.

Probably one of the most universal thoughts ever thought at a time of grief is "How can the world go on as if nothing has happened?" It was somehow reassuring that it didn't. Not only did cars slow down, they pulled off the road. Every single car. Kids riding bikes stopped. One man raking fresh-cut grass took off his hat and nodded to us as we rode by.

Our children were the first to notice all this. It made a remarkable impression on them, this silent tribute, paid out of tradition and respect to someone these people did not even know. We began to watch them with the same curious mixture of emotions that they were watching us.

What were they thinking as we went by? Was it that they might be the next to die, like the old childhood jingle suggests? Were they looking around for a clue, silently wondering who it was underneath the spray of lilies and Christmas ferns?

It wasn't just in the notes of sympathy, the wordless hugs, the tears of sad joy we shared with family that we found comfort and renewal. We found it in these silent strangers outside the car windows.

Especially when a little child in a red pickup shyly raised up two fingers and pressed them against the rear window. She said it all. In the final analysis, it is the bottom line of all our prayers, whoever and wherever we are:

"Peace."

DAUGHTERS WHO CARE TOO MUCH

Sometimes you wonder where talk-show hosts dig up such weird guests. I've not led a completely sheltered life, but I've never met anyone who thinks she is Cleopatra, and I never realized there were such things as men who used to be women married to women who used to be men.

Last week, I read where Sally Jessy Raphael was featuring "daughters embarrassed by their mothers' appearance or behavior."

Now that I can relate to.

I didn't catch the show, but Raphael probably had a run on eligible mother-daughter pairs. In fact, I don't know a mother worth the title who hasn't made her daughter's eyes roll heavenward at some point. Probably lots of points.

My own daughters stayed mortified for

years at a time. How did I embarrass them? Let me count the ways:

They lived in dread that I would actually open my mouth and say something when driving car pool. Mothers were to be seen and not heard.

"Just hush up and drive, Mom," their squinty eyes screamed whenever I cleared my throat to speak.

When I refused to start the engine until everyone was buckled in, they died of embarrassment. When I was late, they died of embarrassment. When I was early, they died of embarrassment. Even when I was on time, just the fact that I was there was embarrassing.

They sought sympathy from their friends when I refused to let them wear boxer shorts to the church picnic. When I said no to getting their ears pierced, they would have put themselves up for adoption if given half a chance.

"You cannot pierce your ears until you are 12," I said.

According to them, I was the only mother in captivity who hadn't taken her daughter down to the jewelry store when they were still in Pampers.

But all these were mere skirmishes compared with the embarrassment over getting their driver's licenses.

Or, actually, not getting them until they actually learned to drive.

The rule in our house was that you had to learn to drive a gearshift car well enough to take the test in it. None of this jumping out of bed on their 16th birthdays and, after a lucky turn around the block with some sleepy policeman, being let loose on the highway.

Getting an old, asthmatic Volkswagen stick shift to behave tends to make one a more careful driver. It's hard to scratch off on a hill, and you have to slow down around curves if you want to keep from stalling. Poor babies. While all their friends (to hear them talk) had brand new fire-engine-red cars of their very own, they had to stay in my good graces so they could borrow a dirty gray Dasher that smelled like dog breath and didn't even have power steering.

It wasn't just my behavior that embarrassed them. My appearance brought them gobs of shame. All I had to do was appear.

My notes on the backs of their report cards were embarrassing. Trimming the crust off their sandwiches, practicing with them on how to shake hands and look people in the eye — everything was embarrassing.

Showing up for Mother's Day at school was embarrassing. Not showing up was embarrassing.

For years I made their lives miserable no matter what I wore. In my fake-leopard-fur-coat stage, they said I looked like Tammy Bakker. In my black boots, they said I looked like an aging, overweight Barbie.

It's a wonder they survived me.

Just the other day, our youngest, home from college for the weekend, was leaving to drive back when I saw that old familiar look again: eyeballs rolled back, hands on hips, a long "Oh-Mom" leaving her limp, and tapping her foot.

All I said was "Don't you think you need a coat? Promise you'll not go over 60. I cut you some oranges to snack on in the car. When was the last time you changed your oil? Are you sure you aren't catching a cold? How much sleep are you getting? Did you balance your checkbook? Have you written your thank-you notes? All that loud music will ruin your ears, and call us when you get there."

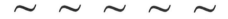

"The best way to keep children home is to make the home atmosphere pleasant — and let the air out of the tires." — Dorothy Parker

MOVING MOUNTAINS: A LOVE STORY

Oh, the things we do for love.
Especially for the love of children.
Even when they are no longer children.

After a summer internship in Los Angeles, teaching in an elementary school in Watts, our daughter is moving to Texas, where she is teaching fourth grade in inner-city Houston. I try to tell myself she's a grown woman on a challenging adventure and that I should just bug off with the lectures and trust the good Lord.

But after so many years of practice, it's hard to give up worrying. I do it so well.

"Mom," she said on the phone from L.A. 10 days ago, "I can't come home before I have to be at work. How am I getting my stuff from Knoxville to Houston?"

So last Saturday I drove out of our driveway, pulling the largest trailer the folks at U-Haul would allow behind a Blazer, and headed for the setting sun.

It's easy to get philosophical on a two-day trip alone on the interstate. Especially when every mile you click off is one more between you and your daughter's new life in an X-rated section of the fourth-largest city in the country.

See how good I am at worrying?

The mileposts flew by almost as fast as the years had. Here I was moving her out, when it hadn't been that long since we brought her home. We'd carried her and all her worldly goods in one arm that happy morning 23 summers ago.

My trip to Houston turned out to be a kind of pilgrimage. As I made my way down from the mountains of Tennessee, through the swamps and soupy heat of Alabama, Mississippi and Louisiana, into the flatlands of Texas, I did a lot of thinking about mothers and daughters and how we really grow up together.

About what it means to have and to hold, and then to let go.

When I got to Houston (crime capital of the nation, hush my mouth), I had a sore bottom and a full heart. It wasn't a lonely trip. Changing voices and a head full of memories kept me company. My Arthur Rubinstein tapes — combined with the way the sun ran along beside me, tagging the rocks and changing greens from chartreuse to olive — made the drive from Knoxville to Gadsden almost like a worship service.

Public radio's Madam Butterfly got me through the loops and belts around Birmingham.

Chet Atkins made it impossible to dwell on gas fumes and the hypnotic march of orange construction drums from Tuscaloosa to Meridian, where every stretch of road is being worked on. Or needs to be.

At Hattiesburg, the sky turned pewter and rain bounced like marbles thrown against the windshield. I was a lost spaceship traveling through an alien silver sea, but I didn't go crazy. I went to South Africa with Wilbur Smith, thanks to the blessed miracle of Books-On-Tape.

After a while, I got used to the do-si-dos that U-Hauls and Blazers do when they go over a bump at 60 mph. Green signs popped up like flashcards, setting into motion memories of other times and places: Lumberton, Miss., became Lumberton, N.C., where a cousin and I used to swim in the caramel-colored waters of the Lumber River. A dead armadillo on the side of the road brought to mind my brother's wedding in Amarillo a thousand years ago, before the wheelchair and the divorce.

A warning outside Baton Rouge reminded me of life's little ironies: "BRIDGE ICES BEFORE ROADS" — the letters of the sign wiggling in the hot, liquid air. Nat King Cole sang about dancing in the dark just as the sky over Lake Charles turned to coal and the radio sent out tornado warnings.

And, all the while, every time I looked up, I saw the words "ysae edam gnivoM" . . . "Moving made easy" . . . the U-Haul slogan, written backward on my rearview mirror.

It is an upside down, backward feeling — letting go, moving on. Motherhood's not-alone, lonely trip. Two things I'll try to remember from this un-hitching:

How the flowers along the side of the road trembled when the big trucks blew past, but they survived. None was uprooted.

And that a mother's love is like kudzu. It follows you everywhere. Even to the crime capital of the world.

~ ~ ~ ~ ~

Here is a breakdown of "father concerns" as compared with "mother concerns."

This comes from a study done by Drs. Gunnard B. Stickler and Daniel D. Breughton. They sound like ivy-tower types, but see if you think they might have something here:

When it comes to raising children, fathers worry about — in this order: 1) finances, 2) health, 3) accidents, 4) discipline, 5) bringing them up "right", 6) drugs, 7) school performance.

Mothers worry most about: 1) health, 2) accidents, 3) bringing them up "right", 4) discipline, 5) drugs, 6) finances, 7) eating right.

ON KNOWING THE SCORE

Once upon a time, there was a little boy who did not like to play basketball.

I know that's hard to believe, but it's true. I know that kid very, very well. Or, at least, as well as a mother can know her own.

His name was, is, George.

George enjoyed going to basketball games, but spent most of the time looking under seats for cups to stomp or making paper airplanes out of the program. In the final moments of the SEC games, when everybody else had their noses pressed half an inch from the TV, George didn't even look up, so engrossed he'd be in gluing the thousandth tiny piece on a one-sixteenth-scale model helicopter.

He loved going to the school gym, squeaking his tennis shoes across the court in different musical patterns or trying out new ape calls to echo up in the rafters.

But he did not like basketball.

One day his mother was at the grocery store, and all she heard was whose son was on what team at the YMCA. The whole world seemed to be abuzz with basketball.

Her best friend's son — who'd just turned 7 — was riding in his mother's cart, wearing a shiny new XXXXXXS undershirt and new tube socks that reached all the way up to his chin.

"He's a Panther," his mother said, patting him proudly on the head. "Center forward . . . a little winner, aren't you, son? A real winner."

Well, you can imagine how George's mother felt. After paying for the baking soda, vinegar and red food coloring George needed for the volcano he was building in the backyard sandbox, she went straight home to talk to him about basketball. He was folded up in his beanbag chair and was teaching the dog to smile.

"How would you like to play basketball?" she said in that singsong voice that sends kids immediately into a coma and, before George knew it, he was a Panther.

Things went pretty well at first, although George concentrated more on learning how to imitate the buzzer than how to double-pump a shot. His favorite part of the game was getting sliced up orange sections to squirt on the girls. Then came the big game with the Saber-toothed Tigers, a team that seemed to have as much trouble as the Panthers in dribbling and keeping their britches up at the same time. Everyone said it would be an "important" game. And it was.

George's mother screamed until she was hoarse and nearly fainted when her son — her son! — kept the other team from getting the ball in the final second. George had been stuffing the silver wrapper off a piece of Juicy Fruit back into the paper to make a fake piece to give his sister, not a clue as to what was happening anywhere else on the court, when suddenly he looked up and saw a herd of Tigers coming at him. Reflexes kicked in. He raised his hand . . . and caught the ball.

Not because he wanted it, he explained later, but simply to keep it from knocking his head off.

"Who won?" he asked on the way home.

"Who won??? YOU won. Because of you, the other team lost!"

"It did?" George said, looking sick. "Ohhhh, noooooo."

"You're a hero, son!"

"No, I'm not. I don't even care about basketball. That guy Jamie . . . the one who would've scored if it hadn't been for me . . . cried last week when they lost."

George was quiet for a long time.

"Next time," he said quietly, "I'm moving out of the way."

That night the laces were taken out of the basketball shoes and used to hang model planes from the ceiling. The Panther shirt was stuffed and reincarnated as the top of the scarecrow in a homespun production of "The Wizard of Oz." Every once in a while, his mom would rant and rave about nobody playing with the expensive basketball they bought for him, but her heart wasn't in it.

She got her money's worth from that basketball. It taught her that she's got herself a winner.

A real winner.

PHONE TAG AND OTHER FAMILY GAMES

Mom, where are you? I have GOT to talk to you!"

It was our daughter's voice. She sounded right pitiful. Said she'd been trying for DAYS and all she got were four rings and a *Hello, we can't come to the phone right now, but . . .*

Kids don't realize that when they leave home, they lose a Mom and gain a Radio Shack Duofone. It has been a busy week, and I love having the kids call home, but at least it gave me a chance to get even for the Telephone Nightmare of '77 — a story our family still laughs about.

I'd been called out of town suddenly on a family emergency. Weekends aren't the best time to leave the preacher's kids — George, then 9, McNair, 8, and Claire, 5 — home alone with their father.

I have a collect call for anyone from Mrs.

Hughs. Will you accept the charges?

"She's not here." It was Claire.

(Louder) *I have a call from Mrs. Hughs. Will you pay?*

(Louder) "She's not here."

Is there anyone older at home?

"Well, my brother's here, but he's been sent to his room for spitting at me . . ."

Is there a baby-sitter?

"No, ma'am. See, dad's just gone for two seconds to the church and he wanted to get one, but the dog ate a pack of crayons and threw up on the baby-sitter list my mom had left by the phone . . . it was all different colors . . . "

Hello, I'm sorry but . . .

"Operator, just cancel the call."

I have a collect call for anyone from Mrs. Hughs. Will you pay for the call?

"She's still not here." It was Claire again.

Is your father there?

"No, ma'am. He's at Arby's fixin' lunch."

Will you pay for the call?

"How much?"

"Operator, that's my little girl . . . Hello? Claire? Just say yes, Claire."

"Do I have to pay out of my own money?"

"Just say yes, Claire."

"Oh, all right. YES."

"Thank you, operator."

"Thank me, mom. I'm paying, remember."

"Thank you. Is everybody OK?"

"Well, George has a fever and just lies there moaning on top of all the Monopoly money, and . . ."

"How much fever?"

"We don't know. He stuck the thermometer in his mashed potatoes and it blew up."

"Tell dad to call me the minute he gets back."

"Oh, wait. Dad said to ask you if you knew where McNair was?"

"WHAT? Is she missing?"

"Well, sort of. She went over to somebody's house and dad

forgot."

"Forgot what?"

"Whose house."

I have a collect call for anyone from Mrs. Hughs. Will you accept the charges?

"Uhmmmmmmm. Well, uh, see."

Is there anyone older at home?

"Well, yes, but he's reading the Bible and doesn't want to be disturbed." It was McNair, thank goodness. "I'll be 9 in July. Is that old enough?"

Ma'am, go ahead.

"How did dad find you?"

"He talked to everybody he'd ever heard of, but by then Jennifer's mother called dad to say they were all ready to go to bed."

"Is George OK? Where's Claire?"

"George is under the bed. Dad said he HAD to have his temperature taken, but there's only the fanny kind left since he broke the other one, and George says he's never felt better in his life . . . Claire is in the kitchen eating Crisco and jelly sandwiches."

"What? Eating what?"

"It's great! Better than peanut butter."

"Go in there right now and tell her to stop."

"Mom, have you ever tried it? . . . 'Don't be such a picky eater,' remember?"

"What did dad have for supper?"

"A can of Beanie-Weenies, a Snickers and a grape soda . . . "

The phone company has a slogan, something to the effect that calling home is the next best thing to being there.

Sometimes it's even better.

LOSING TRACK OF TIME

I t is hard to believe I am old enough to have a mother who is 80.

My mother says it's hard to believe she's old enough to have a daughter who is 50. But while we were busy doing other things, time took us both by surprise and here we are, blowing out 130 candles between us.

My mother doesn't look 80. Or act it, whatever that means. How is one supposed to act at 80? I don't feel 50. But, then, the only 50-year-old I have ever turned inside out is myself. Maybe no 50-year-old has ever felt like they are supposed to feel. I don't know. All I know is that somewhere along the line, invisible parts have been put on hold.

Mother says she doesn't think of herself as being any different than she was at 40. As for me, I look in the mirror and the picture doesn't go with what is on the inside. It's like we are two different people, she and I, staring at each other over the bathroom sink: one, a 50-year-old thing with old jokes and good times written around the eyes, and the laws of gravity pulling away at cheeks and chin.

My face is melting.

Inside, underneath, within is another person, a prisoner of time, refugee of 50 heart-shaped, February birthday cakes. I hardly recognize the face in the mirror. Behind the sag and wrinkles is the same old me, without the new old face. It's scary.

If you stop and think about it — which I really don't very often, but turning half a century old does make one breathe deeply and try to figure out what is going on — you begin to realize that time makes us strangers to ourselves, and sometimes to those we love.

I don't live near my mother, and I see her only two or three times a year, a fact of life that will soon repeat itself as my own children move on to make homes of their own in other places. Each time I see my mother, it's a new shock that she looks older or takes it slower.

Time may heal most wounds, but it also creates a few of its own.

Age made my mother-in-law, in many ways, a stranger to herself and to those of us who loved her. Before her death, her mind darted in and out of current reality. She remembered every detail of Irwinton, Ga., just as it was when she was 13 and drove the first car anyone ever drove down its one dirt road. Yet she sometimes had trouble figuring out who I was or why our youngest child — her namesake — was not the baby she imagined crying in the next room.

She remembered who lived in what house all up and down the neighborhood in Moultrie, Ga., where she raised her sons and looked after her own mother-in-law until time won out, as it always does. But she could no longer take care of herself. Mercifully, her mind painted over the strange, lonely world to which that "ever-flowing stream" had taken her. She set her clock backward, returning to be once again with the people and in the places she knew best and loved most.

There was no "we" or "us" any longer for her. Not since her husband of fifty-plus years died two springs before her. But she preferred to live in a corner of her mind to which the sad news hadn't yet come.

One day when our daughter Claire was about 4, she asked me what it had been like on the ark.

"I wasn't on the ark!" I told her, jotting down a reminder to get some Oil of Olay or a face-lift.

"Then why didn't you drown?"

Today as I turn 50, I feel like maybe I was on the ark and just don't remember.

There are so many things I can't remember. My father died when I was pregnant with our first child, 24 years ago. Time has marched across my memories of him, leaving some intact and taking others out with the tide.

I remember the stories of the Laughing Man he told as we lay in the hammock after supper at the beach long, long years ago. But I had forgotten the letter he wrote me when I turned 16, until I found it the other night in a stack of old papers.

Never in a million years did I think I would ever forget what each of my own children looked like at 6 or 10 or the first time I saw them in the hospital. Now I have to take the pictures out of the album and look on the back to check my hunches.

So, what does it feel like to turn 50? Or 80? Or 90?

It's a little bit like drowning.

A FAMILY'S BEST FRIEND

Thisis a talking dog story. It's for everyone who doesn't believe in miracles — and for those who are grateful for them.

Actually, talking dogs aren't all that unusual. Most people whose pets are people can vouch for the fact that the family member who happens to be a dog can speak volumes over the years.

Knuckles started talking early on.

Sixteen years ago this summer, my husband and our three children stood over a litter of squirming, 6-week-old Lhasa apsos, trying to decide which one to take home. Lhasas are a shrink-art version of an Old English sheep dog. As puppies, they look more like something you'd powder your face with or use to get the cobwebs off the ceiling than something you bring home and love your whole life long.

Over in the corner that day was the smallest, the scrawniest, the runtiest little thing you ever saw. He took one look at our kids, opened his brown saucer eyes and said, "Hi, guys. You can stop looking now. I'm all yours."

It was Knuckles.

On the way home, son George and his dad discussed what to name the new baby. They'd just about decided on Captain Crunch when Knuckles scrunched up his rear end, took as deep a breath as his tiny lungs would allow and did a flying leap from his shoe box into George's lap.

"Hey, Dad!" George said. "He's just the size of your knuckles."

Knuckles smiled, thanked them for not naming him off a cereal box and snored peacefully all the way home.

The children each donated a stuffed animal to keep the new puppy company, and the next morning Knuckles' bed was such a mass of animal stuffings, it was hard to tell where make-believe ended and reality began.

Over the years, Knuckles has had a lot to say to our family.

There was the time we took him camping, and Knuckles got so excited about seeing his reflection in the creek he leaned over and fell in. One by one the children jumped in after him, which would have been one thing if it had been sunny July instead of nearly Thanksgiving, when your teeth chattered even when you were fully clothed and standing on dry land.

The children were hysterical, thinking that Knuckles might have been swept away had they not been there to save him. It took every towel in the tent and a long discussion about dog heaven to get everyone dry and warm.

That was the night Knuckles talked me out of Dog Rule No. 1. From then on — until she left for college — Knuckles slept with our daughter Claire. Not just in the same room. In the same bed. Under the covers. With his head on her pillow.

Rule No. 2 was about food. My job was to feed people. I didn't "do" dogs. Until the night of the Green Noodle Casserole. I refuse to repeat the names my family called that casserole when I put it on the table, but by the time they were finished describing it, it was stone-cold. Even the garbage disposal struggled with it, but Knuckles, bless his heart, looked up and said, "What do they know? You're such a good cook . . . Mind if I have a bite?"

He liked it so much his eyes watered.

In his 16 years with us, Knuckles has been baby-sitter, best friend, confidant, watchdog, playmate. He's gone down the steps with the children on Christmas morning, written them at camp, watched them pack for college. He's remembered birthdays and anniversaries and sat at his master's feet way into the night at tax time, breathing quiet little sighs of sympathy.

His favorite spot was at the back door, waiting to hear a car pull up or a bike screech to a halt.

Monday he made his final trip in the family car. His health had deteriorated to the point that he had to be lifted up steps, carried in and out. Even then, he whimpered in pain.

Our daughter McNair and her father bought him two scoops of his favorite kind of ice cream before putting him gently down on the table at the vet's. They patted him. Thanked him. Remembered with him. And stayed with him until it was over.

I don't know what you're supposed to say at dog funerals. I've mostly muffled my way through goldfish and hamster burials, but I know that Knuckles has said a lot to us over the years about what it means to be a family and to care for someone else, to be faithful and funny, loyal and loved.

His voice will always be a part of who we are.

FREEZE FRAME

Last week when I blew out the candle on my birthday cake, it occurred to me that I am the same age my father was the year he died.

As I drew in breath to make my wish, a picture of my father sitting at the piano flashed up on the screen in my head.

My family was smart enough not to put but one candle on my cake — a frozen yogurt affair with nondairy topping and a swear-to-it disclaimer about saturated fats. Fifty-two candles would probably set off the smoke detector.

Everyone said my father was a young man when he died. I didn't believe it then, but I sure believe it now. I was 25, just a few months younger than our oldest child is now, the night my father collapsed in the driveway of his house in Richmond, Va. Without warning. We had both been to church: He'd been the speaker at a Thanksgiving week worship service at his church in Richmond; I had been at a Sunday school planning session at my church in Norfolk, Va., some three hours away by car.

We didn't have answering machines then, so my brothers and sisters took turns trying to reach me. When I heard my brother Jimmy's voice on the other end of the phone . . . "You need to sit down; I have something to tell you" . . . I thought it was going to be good news. Those were the birthing years for our family. I was due in six months. My sister-in-law had just called a week before to say she was pregnant. Here was Jimmy with news.

"News" in those days did not mean "death."

Perhaps if my father had known to stick to yogurt cakes, had put out his cigarettes earlier, I wouldn't have gotten that phone call. Or if he had been born in time for bypass surgery that could have saved his life, like it did my brother Bobby's life in 1978.

Two things saved Bobby's life: the fact that he was in a duck blind with three doctor friends when it happened, and the new technology waiting for him when the air ambulance got to Duke Medical Center. Daddy wasn't so lucky.

We consoled ourselves, or tried to, by saying he would have been miserable had he been "revived." He never regained consciousness. There had been brain loss. If they had gotten his heart started again, it would have meant a pins-and-needles life. Not his style.

When the organ played "For All the Saints Who From Their Labors Rest" at his funeral, my mother leaned over the five of us and said, "He doesn't want to REST!"

Resting is certainly not something he was very good at.

Fishing was. He often took me along, but I always felt sorry for the fish and, as soon as I could get away with it, would drag my fingers in the water and spend the rest of the afternoon asking him hard questions.

The kind adults are supposed to know the answers to.

He was also good at the piano. He never seemed to want to play the hymns the way they'd been written. He always jazzed them up. Added a little ragtime. He was good at baseball, at telling jokes, and he had a look about him that made your feet itch with shame should he catch you in a lie or a cuss word or the makings of a sassy answer.

There is enough of him in me to know now that his answers were, like mine are, bought and paid for by hard thinking, a hopeful faith and a belief that sometimes all we can do is to play our hunches. I don't even have a piano anymore, but I hope my theology, like his, has a nice dance rhythm to it.

Maybe it's old age that makes these scenes so sharp in my mind. The advice I hear over and over from those piano lessons and fishing trips is "think for yourself." I wonder how he would feel should he know my answers sometimes take me upstream, pulling me against the current of orthodoxy or tradition. He might not agree, but I think he would understand.

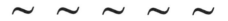

> *Dad, how many stars are there in the sky?*
> "I don't know."
> *Dad, who invented ketchup?*
> "I don't know."
> *Dad, when do worms sleep?*
> "I don't know."
> *Dad, I hope you don't mind me asking all these questions.*
> "Of course not, son. How else will you learn anything?"

SISTERS AND 'BOTHERS'

Oh, God," the little girl said in her prayers one night, "I know you're supposed to love everybody, but are you sure you've met my brother?" If you are lucky, you can understand those words.

I probably would never have had the nerve to actually sell my brothers into slavery, like Joseph's did in the Old Testament. But having grown up in a big family, I'd have been tempted if the opportunity had come up at the right time.

Like the time my brother had 50 Red Top baby chicks delivered to my dorm, C.O.D.

It's hard for me to imagine what it would be like not to have had a big brother or a big sister. Nobody to stick up for you, to tease you, to get you out of trouble. To explain the real facts of life.

There's a dimension to brotherhood and

sisterhood found in no other relationship. Teamwork, acceptance, identity — all scrambled up in genes and proximity. Lucky for me, I got a lot of practice in close encounters of the family kind. Two brothers and two sisters. But like most good things in life, we don't fully appreciate what we have.

Back then, families actually ate together. Good for your morale, but bad on your shins if you happen to sit directly across from two older brothers who kick you under the table, trying to get you to complain so they can call you a tattletale.

Every morning we had family prayers. I never closed my eyes. If I did, my brother Jimmy would poke a hole in my egg or snitch my cinnamon toast. Bobby used to bet me I couldn't keep my eyes open without blinking while Daddy read from the Bible. Even if my eyeballs had exploded all over the table . . . even if the angel Gabriel had swooped down and commanded me to BLINK! . . . I would not have done it.

Have you ever tried not to blink during the story of the creation? I am sure my parents thought I was having some kind of religious experience.

If my Sunday school teachers had ever asked me why I wanted to go heaven, I'd have told them, "Because I know my brothers will not be there." Now I fudge on grocery money so I can talk to them whenever I get lonely or bored or just feel like it.

But don't tell them I said that.

The Bible tells us we're supposed to honor our father and mother. Brothers and sisters have to earn it — through marathon games of Monopoly and hide-and-seek, long talks late into the night over bags of potato chips while the rest of the world nods off.

Probably the best compliment we can pay our parents is to strengthen the ties that bind us to our brothers and sisters, even after our room is cleaned out and all our stuffed animals go to flea markets.

Even — no, especially — after our parents are gone.

COMINGS AND GOINGS

But, Mom, this is what aunts and uncles do . . . not children."

My daughter and I are talking very long-distance on the phone about last-minute Thanksgiving plans. She's telling me what time her plane is getting in and asking when the others will arrive. I've just told her that her brother might not make it until dinnertime Thursday because he has to work until 10 Wednesday night, and it's a six-hour drive.

Her sister gets in late Wednesday from college but has warned everyone that exams start the day she gets back, so she's spending the weekend with her philosophy syllabus.

Thanksgiving is not what it used to be at our house, back when everybody had the same ZIP code, and, if we wanted to "reach out and touch" each other, we didn't have to do it by phone.

The torch is being passed, as they say, and Thanksgiving is one of those times that the matches get struck. In even the closest-knit of families the time comes when you need to drop a stitch for the pattern to come out right. Children who are given roots, but no wings, are to be pitied. My family never made me feel guilty or that it was inappropriate somehow for me not to come home when the tides shifted and the currents of life took me in other directions.

Our daughter remembers phone conversations in the background of her 23 other Thanksgivings, conversations her father and I had with our parents and brothers and sisters about whether we would be "going home" for Thanksgiving.

"I can't imagine," she says, sounding very far away, "not coming home, or George and Claire being somewhere else for the holidays."

But a round-trip ticket from Houston on a first-year teacher's salary (or any teacher's salary, for that matter) takes a big bite out of the budget and is hard to rationalize when Christmas is just weeks away.

I know how she feels.

To me, Thanksgiving used to mean my mother's ambrosia, my father's blessing and a marathon game of Monopoly with brothers, sisters and assorted cousins. That was then and this is now, and in between came all the cutting and hemming, the letting out a seam here, taking in a tuck there that goes into the fabric of our lives.

With time, Thanksgiving meant my mother's ambrosia, my father's blessing and midterms instead of Monopoly. Then, one week before Thanksgiving when I was pregnant with our first child — and plans had already been made to gather — my father had a heart attack. Had I known the Thanksgiving before that it would be the last time I would ever hear his blessing at the table, I would have listened closer.

Then came the years of making my own ambrosia and swapping Monopoly for diapers . . . lopsided paper turkeys taped to the fridge . . . school plays that had us clapping until our hands stung over a fourth-grade Pilgrim.

Now, here I am talking to that pilgrim a thousand miles from home, and she's telling me something we both know from experience.

Thanksgiving is one of those rites-of-passage times. High-water marks in the ever-flowing stream of time:

The first Thanksgiving home after going to college, and the shock that comes with being so ready to come home . . . but after the ambrosia, the loads of laundry, the late-night talk over cold dressing and turkey sandwiches . . . so ready to leave.

The first Thanksgiving as a part of someone else's family. Maybe they put marshmallows in their ambrosia, or never heard of ambrosia, and even if you do play Monopoly, sending your new father-in-law to jail isn't as much fun as sending a cousin.

Then, before you know it, you're standing in the kitchen talking with adult children whose Thanksgivings are out of your control.

It's funny, isn't it?

And sad.

And frightening.

But, because of who they've become and what's out there waiting for them, and because of some mysterious time clock that, thank goodness, God puts in every child's and parent's heart . . . it is also wonderful in a grown-up kind of way.

V. WONDERS OF HEAVEN AND EARTH

It is Saturday. I have just spent the morning at the beauty parlor, getting highlights to cover the gray. Then, would you believe, I spent the afternoon lying in the sun in my backyard, trying to get a tan.

I am telling you all this just in case you don't know that I am not to be trusted when it comes to thinking logically. Here I am, trying to lighten my hair and darken my skin. Doesn't make sense, does it?

Sometimes, though, life doesn't make a whole lot of sense. Sometimes we have to put our brains on hold and grab the moment. Not think so much, just accept the wonder of it all. Sometimes we need to forget all we have been told and all we know — and look around for something new to happen.

Don't tell my children I said all this.

SOAKIN' UP
THE MOUNTAINS

I n his book on growing up in Cades Cove, Randolph Shields tells how his grandmother used to sit in her rocking chair on the porch for hours at a time, staring off into space.

"What are you doing, Grandma?"

"Ah, just settin' here, soakin' in the mountains."

There's no better place to watch the dance of life and death than the mountains — and no better time than when fall comes for its annual visit in Cades Cove.

From June until August, the park service closes the road through Cades Cove every Saturday morning until 10, allowing bikers and hikers the peaceful, quiet, exhaust-fumeless pleasure of "soakin' in" the summer magic of that place. I've spent a dozen summer mornings walking the loop, sponging up the sights and smells, counting my blessings that God had the brilliant idea to create places like Cades Cove and folks in Tennessee had the sense to preserve it.

There are only a couple of bikers and no other hikers the morning a friend and I decided to race the sun as it stretches and yawns its way over to Cades Cove. It is my last Cades Cove pilgrimage before winter sets in.

We get there at first light, driving the hour-long trip to the Cades Cove parking lot in sleepy silence, except for the occasional squeak of plastic-on-plastic as we take our Pilot coffee cups in and out of their holders.

Outside Townsend, we slide Ray Lynch into the car tape deck and listen to his "star music" as we ride the curves through the park.

The headlights catch the leaves as they jitterbug across the road, and when a passing Winnebago stirs up a whirlwind of reds and browns and crispy maroons, the world outside the car windows turns into a kaleidoscope.

" . . . *'As dry leaves before the hurricane fly,'* " I think to myself, buttoning the top button of my windbreaker.

What a perfect image. As we ride our sleigh through a leaf storm in the almost-frosty air, Old Man Winter — if not Saint Nick — seems close on our heels.

And it is kind of like Christmas, when, what to our wondering eyes, the whole world seems a gift, full of surprises:

Wild turkeys (I guess they were wild) play a game of ring-around-the-rosie behind a clump of joe-pye weed.

Blue asters bob and bend in the rustling grass.

A raccoon jay-runs across our path.

We stop counting deer after we get to 50.

Every time I go to Cades Cove in the early morning, I see something new. This time it was — what? a weasel? a ferret? — something bigger than a chipmunk and smaller than a fox and definitely not a squirrel. It looked at me and I looked at it, and neither one could figure out exactly what we'd come across.

Unfortunately, it gave up and ran off too soon.

We decided to cut through Sparks Lane, and the sun came up as we sloshed through the spillway across Maple Branch, lighting up the mica underwater and double-exposing the Queen Anne's lace stitched along the creek bed.

Just as rough weather makes good timber, a coming storm can turn a normal sunrise into teeth-chattering beauty.

The last mile of the loop, it began to rain.

Sunlight, soaked up in the mist of passing night and the first drops of a settling-in rain, hung like prisms off the branches of trees overhead. For a moment, nothing else in the whole world mattered.

No wonder Jesus wants us to be sunbeams.

It has taken almost 52 years to get the real meaning of that old Bible school song.

But now I understand why.

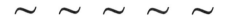

Art Linkletter, Pied Piper of the kindergarten set, is probably best known for getting kids to say "the darndest things." He would no doubt enjoy Stuart Hample and Eric Marshall's compilation of "Children's Letters to God," found in most bookstores.

Out of the mouths of babes come some 50 burning questions and comments, illustrated with appropriate childlike drawings. What they ask God ranges from lispy cute to cutting-edge theology: In Bible times, did they really talk that fancy? It's OK that you made different religions, but don't you get mixed up sometimes? How come you did all those miracles in the old days and don't do any now?

All this reminds me of the best translation I ever heard of the trespasser line in the Lord's Prayer. The theologian in this case was about 5:

It means "forgive us our trash baskets as we forgive those who put trash in our baskets."

MOON MADNESS

Get ready for a full moon tonight. Wish away the clouds so we can see it, feel it. Even talk to it, if we've any of the poet in us.

From T.S. Eliot to James Bond, from Plato to Charlie Brown, philosophers, writers and others have worked under its spell, calling it a vast wasteland, a circumambulating aphrodisiac, the mistress of melancholy, a ghostly galleon tossed upon cloudy seas.

Full moons are not only light bulbs for writers and thinkers. They give us simpler folks something to celebrate.

They are for howling, for high tides, for hanky-panky.

A night for going out of your mind.

It took us $30 billion to travel a quarter of a million miles to actually shake hands with the Man in the Moon. Frank Borman, broadcasting from Apollo VIII on Christmas Eve 1968, echoed what cavemen and other poets concluded long ago: The moon is a different thing to each person. A forbidding place. Lonely and expansive.

Heat, cold, craters of silence.

At the time, it represented a kind of new Jerusalem. Four days after the first moon landing, President Nixon said, "This is the greatest week in the history of the world since the creation."

It's easy to get carried away when it comes to the moon.

Whether you're a cat with a fiddle, a sleepy-time threesome in a wooden shoe, a vampire or Andy Williams in search of a top hit, the moon is full of magic.

It's the earth's timepiece. At its bidding, the seas rise and fall — great swells of breath that spill out over the rocks and sands of time and place.

By it, the sun sets its clocks, plans its paint jobs, plays its daily games of show and tell. Some say even the stork schedules his routes according to what the moon is up to.

Moonlight, like moonshine, is intoxicating.

I remember watching it paddle across the sky through rippling pine trees the long night I spent in a sleeping bag as a Brownie Scout on my first camping trip. I was too scared to close my eyes, too homesick to sleep, too cold to get up and tell my leader. I decided then and there that no matter how old I got, what awful and wonderful things happened to me or how far from home I eventually went, I would never forget the night the moon and I kept each other company.

It's a promise I have kept.

When I got a little older, my brothers told me about a certain kind of wolf that came out on the full moon and stalked the neighborhood for a little fast food. I made sure no part of my body hung off the bed, tempting any wolf slinking out of my closet or up from the basement . . . where, said my brothers, wolves are apt to hide.

Long after I learned there were no such things, I still took precautions. You can't be too careful.

I've watched men walk on the moon. I've eaten my share of Moon Pies. Been moonstruck a time or two. I've looked at the moon through sea oats and telescopes, from backseats of cars and out of airplane windows.

I've seen it lying like a coverlet on a sleeping ocean.

I've seen it stuck like a slice of lemon on the teacup of the world.

I've seen its Cheshire-cat grin, its pumpkin face, its bloodshot eyes.

No matter what phase it's in or what mood I am in, it brings a kind of mesmerizing mystery into my life.

Cows jump over it. Musicians turn it into a sonata or a river. Add to it a sixpence, and they say your dreams come true.

Neither scientist nor psalmist can quite figure it out.

Once I saw the moon in a time warp. A freeze-frame from creation. I could almost touch it. Millions of years slipped away, and it was the way it had been in the beginning. Before God had flung out the stars to keep it company.

It happened the night a friend and I went on a midnight walk through Four Hole Swamp in the Francis Beidler Forest near Charleston, S.C. The world was a shining piece of mica, black and silver and silent. I saw, without a doubt, what the world looked like long before God moved across the water. Before any seeds were planted. Before the sun rode its chariot across the sky.

Before sonatas and cheese and space shots.

It was a sight no mind or muse could ever, ever unravel.

So.

Take a look outside tonight. Full moons may come like clockwork, but we've lost something important if we think of them as routine.

Remember, though, just to be on the safe side — don't let an arm or leg hang off the bed.

THINGS THAT GO CHIRP IN THE NIGHT

Entomologists tell us that you don't need a thermometer to tell the temperature.

A cricket can do it just as well.

A cricket regulates his/her (Guy? Girl? Can you tell?) chirps according to how hot or cold it is.

Count the number of chirps per minute, divide by four and add 40. The number you come up with corresponds, roughly, to the temperature in degrees Fahrenheit.

According to the cricket trapped somewhere in our kitchen, it is 400 degrees outside. He's been going three days now and I'm so crazy from listening, the number you get after counting chirps has changed from a weather to a mental health report. It's my blood pressure, plus 40.

He never seems to slow down. Don't they ever get tired?

All night. All day.

And it's not "chirp chirp," either. It's more like EEEEEEEEEK EEEEEEEEK. The only time he stops is when we come in the kitchen to listen where the sound is coming from.

I pull out the refrigerator.

No cricket.

I take everything off the shelf in the pantry.

No cricket.

I upside all the bottles and brushes under the sink.

No cricket.

I sweep under all the counters, the chairs, the sills and the doors.

No cricket.

I shake the curtains, jiggle all the plates and saucers, rattle pots and pans.

No cricket.

I give up.

Then, as I am sliding a pan of toast into the oven, I see something move inside the clear plastic dials on the stove.

CRICKET.

There's no way to get him out, short of bashing in the whole thing. I don't think the insurance company would buy that. Whoever heard of a $350 cricket?

What's worse, our cricket has a friend somewhere loose in our house, too.

His friend doesn't say much, but this is a good example of silence speaking louder than words.

His friend is a roach.

Not an ordinary roach, either. It's extra hairy, extra fast and extra big. Having moved here from Charleston, S.C., I know my roaches.

This one is not normal.

The first time I saw him, he was sitting at our breakfast table picking his teeth. The last time I saw him, he was chasing me . . . trying to step on me. If I hadn't jumped up on the bed, he would have mashed me flat.

You'd think a mezzo-soprano cricket and a psychopathic roach would be enough. But no.

We've also got a spider on our back porch with a warped sense of humor.

He's not normal either. His web is made of 3-pound fish line and rubber cement, and it completely covers our back door frame. Every morning, this same spider drops down from the roof and hangs there, waiting for us to go out for the paper.

And every morning we forget.

Going through that thing is like a sideways bungee jump.

Crickets chirp. Roaches charge.

Spiders laugh.

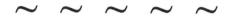

Busy as a bee? Probably not. The average worker bee visits 50-100 flowers each time he buzzes out of the hive. One pound of honey represents 55,000 miles of bee flying time. Even with all that work, a bee gathers only enough nectar to make 1 / 12 of a teaspoon of honey in his lifetime.

SOUVENIRS OF SALVATION

On or about March 27, 1963, at approximately 12:03 a.m. in a first-floor dormitory at Agnes Scott College in Atlanta, Ga., I had a vision.

When I entered my room, there on my desk, next to apple cores and a half-typed World Religions paper, was a lighted cross about six inches tall. It was green with little red drops on it. It slowly turned round and round.

"Becky," I said to my roommate. "Help."

"Huh?" she moaned, pretending to be asleep.

"On my desk over there," I whispered, "Do you see it?"

"See what?"

"It's a . . . it's a . . . "

Well, what it was was a plastic, luminous, battery-operated cross that Becky had gotten in the mail from her aunt. If you held it up to the light for a few minutes, it glowed in the dark. There was a button you pushed to make it turn. The red things were supposed to be drops of blood.

For $2.50 plus postage, Becky and her aunt had scared the curlers out of my hair and put me onto a disturbing fascination for the ever-growing market of religious junk. What one minister friend of mine calls the flotsam and jetsam of faith. Souvenirs of salvation.

That glow-in-the-dark cross, awesome as it was, is kid's play compared to what you can get these days. I hate to think what would have happened if Becky's aunt had sent the thing I saw in a catalog the other day: an electric, near life-size cross on which, when you rub it and pray "the Miracle Prayer," the face of Jesus appears and says a special message just for you. Kind of like a spiritual version of Chatty Cathy.

There are Scripture Checks from Response House, each one perfectly legal, with your choice of Noah's rainbow or a Christian pole vaulter's picture and the verse, "Ask and it will be given you," printed on every check.

My brother — a Presbyterian minister — says he has personally seen a vial of Oral Roberts Evangelistic Association and Abundant Life Prayer Group Holy Oil and a framed picture of Jesus With The Moving Eyes. When it rains, he cries.

Not long ago, I browsed through several Christian bookstores and found:

— New Testament frisbees: "Jesus will give you a lift all the way."

— Applications for a Christian Charm Course.

— 14-carat crown-of-thorns pierced earrings.

— Buttons that say, "I was saved last night" and "I Love You . . . Is That OK?" signed, in cursive, *Jesus Christ.*

— Spiritual fertilizers for house plants: "Fertilize with a green-thumb inspiration" reads the copy for little stakes "impregnated" (I'm quoting off the instructions) with fertilizers and a passage of scripture.

Then there are the bumper stickers:

PREPARE FOR YOUR FINALS: READ THE BIBLE . . . CHRISTIANS HAVE MORE FUN, ESPECIALLY LATER . . . NO

VISITORS ALLOWED IN HEAVEN . . . I'M A FOOL FOR
CHRIST. WHOSE FOOL ARE YOU?

One manufacturer of "Christian Clothing" (can T-shirts get
converted?) makes this pitch: "Buy Christian jerseys because God's
children make unique witnesses when they wear authentic New
Zealand rugby shirts."

Bumper-sticker theology and rinky-dink religious rubbish —
all this stuff — make comic book caricatures of the life and
teachings of Jesus Christ. It trivializes. It demeans.

It squeezes the divine into a dime store.

Fertilizers aren't holy, and Christ doesn't need people to honk
or wave or turn on their windshield wipers to let others know they
love him. I think he is, frankly, a little embarrassed over the
Christian Pet Rock you can buy as a reminder that he is The Rock.

One bookmark I saw said, "God so loved the world, he didn't
send a committee."

Neither did he send a Coney Island trinket seller.

~　~　~　~　~

*"To whom much is given ". . . not as
much is given away. Or, as The Washington
Post puts it: " . . . households with incomes of
less than $10,000 gave twice as much (5.5
percent) of their income to charity as did those
earning $100,000 a year (2.9 percent)."*

WHO'S GOD . . .

God is great, God is good . . ."
An article in Newsweek suggests these words may be more than echoes from childhood. Studies by sociologist-novelist-priest Andrew Greeley indicate that more than half of all Americans pray at least once a day. Seventy-eight percent pray once a week.

The pendulum, it seems, has swung from the "me" generation to the "Thee" generation.

From body to soul.

The current issue of Books in Print lists 2,000 titles on prayer and spiritual growth. Newsweek points out this is more than three times the number of books on the subject of sexual intimacy.

Statistics show that 40 percent of Americans attend religious services once a week, but Greeley says an even more significant "barometer" of our spirituality is the growing number of people who pray seriously, consistently and out of conviction. He gives these run-downs:

— 91% of women pray; 85% of men;

— 94% of blacks; 87% of whites;

— 15% regularly receive "definite" answers to specific prayers; 27% never; 25% "once or twice."

The article discusses the prayer habits of clergy and lay-people from a variety of religious perspectives, including medical doctors who document the positive effect of intercessory prayers for the sick.

The most fascinating result of Greeley's studies is evidence that even atheists pray: Of the 13% of Americans who are atheists or agnostics, "nearly one of five prays daily . . . wagering that there is a God who hears them."

Orson Welles once said that the reason he never prayed was because he didn't want to bore God. That kind of smarty-pants attitude doesn't go over as well today. God may be many things with us, but bored isn't one of them.

If somehow we could listen to our brothers and sisters across town and across the world, I think we would hear the same prayer — from the roughest of us to the most pious: Please make the bad people good and the good people nice.

We differ not in what we want and need. It is our understanding of the voice and reality on the other end of our prayers that divides us, often sadly cutting us off from each other spiritually. The Judeo-Christian tradition says simply that God is love. The Bible compares God with an earthly parent, with wind, light, fire.

But what do we mean when we say God?

Deidre Sullivan proposed to Doubleday Books that she ask that question to people across the United States, and her book gives a bird's-eye view of modern day, grass roots theology. Consider these answers from Sullivan's book, "What Do We Mean When We Say God":

"I think of God (as) the father I never had because my father left my mother when I was 1," says a 12-year-old boy in Anchorage.

"If I am the sail, God is the wind," explains a TV talk show host in New York City. "If I am the roots, God is the tree."

A young mother in New Jersey says God is "that part of us

that cares for a child starving in another country." A freshman at the University of Arkansas describes God as having "a dark complexion, coarse hair and red eyes. He's very handsome."

According to an Illinois architect, "If there is anything you care enough about for which you would give up your life, then you know what God means. Otherwise, forget it."

To school principal Dan Smith, "He's the dad whose lap I've never outgrown." To 16-year-old Lisa Hazen, "Santa Claus comes to mind. I know Santa Claus is not real, but if he was, God would have the exact personality of him."

"Sometimes when I meditate," says a 53-year-old attorney, "God comes up as my grandmother with a frying pan in her hand."

Musician Graham Nash says, "Putting a face on God is a human trick to make Him more accessible."

Film producer Catherine Teague sees "God as the sea. I think of people as bowls by the sea and we sit there and the sea pours into the bowl and it brings whatever it is that we are looking for."

A 77-year-old Unity minister in Laguna Hills, Calif., sums it up this way: "A man without God is like a teenager with a powerful car."

WILL AND WILL NOT

A little boy is leading his horse in from the field to the barn. Something startles the horse. Maybe a leaf falls and tickles the horse's nose. In a split-second reflex action, the horse shies, knocking the little boy to the ground. The boy hits his head on a stone. Weeks later, he's still in a coma.

A family of five on the way to the beach crosses a railroad track and the car is struck by a train. It takes two hours to remove the bodies.

Why them instead of me or you? Or someone who is old and finished with living?

Some people will tell you it is God's will.

I found out today that the teenaged son of a friend of mine has leukemia.

"It sure is hard to understand God's will," said the friend who called to tell me the news, " . . . but God has a reason for this."

Baloney.

A number of years ago, I worked on a story about a woman whose 2-year-old son had fallen off a dock while she was standing next to him. He drowned. She said the hardest part of the whole thing was working through the idea that it had been God's will.

A lot of well-meaning people told her that her anger and despair were unworthy emotions for a Christian because if we read the Bible enough times, if our faith is strong enough, we accept as God's will whatever happens. All we need to do is to screw the lid tighter on the jar of faith. To swallow the sugar-coated, easy-quoted platitudes from old hymns and old testaments.

Is something wrong with people who can't pop platitudes like aspirin for a headache? I don't believe cancer and car accidents, serial killings and pornography are part of God's will. I don't believe in a creator-God who flings out the stars and stomps up the mountains and spits out the seas — and then sets up shop in heaven before a giant control panel, where he begins punching all the buttons, bouncing all the balls and pulling all the plugs:

"Make that leaf fall just in time to startle that particular horse and make the horse twist just this way so his hoof kicks this one boy in that exact crucial spot . . ."

One of the worst things that happens in Christian circles is that some of us point an accusing finger at others of us who can't bandage up our pain by saying these things are some kind of divinely ordained test or punishment.

Didn't that sort of God go out with bongo drums and firstborn bonfires?

Yet, when circumstances deal a death blow, many biblical one-liners are taken out of context: *The Lord giveth and the Lord taketh away, blessed be the name of the Lord.* (Job 1:21); *My people perish for their lack of knowledge.* (Hosea 4:6).

These passages seem to roll off some lips like commercial jingles. I am no biblical scholar, but I am a lie-awake-at-night, middle-aged woman who struggles to square a Christian faith with the events of the day.

What does make sense is the comment a seminary professor made to a young man who was explaining his call into full-time Christian service: "Now I know why God gave me and my wife a retarded child," said the seminarian. "Because of this child, I have been led into the ministry." The professor looked this well-meaning father in the eyes and said, "I really don't believe God needs you that badly."

It just doesn't fit that God cut the blood supply to a boy's brain to get a message across to his father. Albert Einstein once said, "God may be sophisticated, but he's not malicious."

So, what does the minister mean when he prays "if it be thy will, heal . . . or bring peace . . . or help the hungry?" Wouldn't a better word be "since"?

God's will isn't programmed into some heavenly computer. It is brought about by doctors who cure and world leaders who make peace; people who share so others won't starve; those who visit the prisons and look under the rocks of society for people who are hurt or lonely or discarded.

Christ taught us not only to pray that God's will be done, but to do things and be things that help make it happen. Who can look at all the suffering and waste and hate in the world and say that — even in some mysterious way — it is God's will?

Not me.

ON A FIRST-NAME BASIS

My God!"

Yes?

"Huh???"

You called?

"What do you mean, 'You called?'
Who is this?

*God. Your God. That's who you called,
isn't it?*

"Am I on Candid Camera?"

You said, 'My God!' — and here I am.

"Well, I wasn't talking to you exactly."

*Who were you talking to? Yourself? Then
why not use your own name?*

"Look. 'Oh, God' . . . 'My God' . . . 'Good
God' . . . they are all just things you say. I
mean, let's not get so ultimate here. Go back
to . . . to . . . whatever you were doing. I didn't
mean to interrupt. It wasn't very important.
I'm not dying or praying or in deep trouble or
anything like that. Don't worry. I'll let you

know when I need you."

How?

"I'll call you."

You just did.

"I know, but I didn't really mean GOD God. It was just an expression. Like Good Grief!

That's another strange one.

"Don't take it so seriously. People say 'God' this and 'God' that every day, and all they mean in that the soup is too hot or the teacher is giving a test or they missed a putt.

Why not say 'Rats!' or 'Darn it!' Or even 'Oh, Devil!' Wouldn't that fit better?

"It just doesn't have the same ring. OHHH, GOD! . . . That sounds, you know, important."

Yes, I know. It is. That's why I answered.

"I mean, sometimes people say, 'Oh, God,' when something happens to them, and they think it's funny. Like, 'Oh, God, you should have seen her expression.' Or 'God! I love this sweater!' "

Am I supposed to answer back? Do they want advice or comfort or anything from me when they say those things?

"Nah. It's just a figure of speech. Just ignore it."

Hmmmmm. What about God, damn it? I hear that a lot. What do they expect me to do about that?

"Well, nothing, really. They are just joking."

Doesn't sound like it when they say it. To ask God to damn something or somebody is pretty heavy duty, if you stop and think about it. What if I did damn all husbands, wives, bosses, teachers, friends that folks have asked me to?

"Oh, come on. Be a sport. I walk by the desk and hit my knee on the corner and it hurts like God knows what — oops! sorry — and I say, rubbing my knee, 'God, damn . . .' "

You want me to damn the table? The knee? You?

"No. It's just an expression. It makes me feel better."

That's strange because I'm really not into damning. I'm pretty selective about things like that. You humans are much more into the damning thing than I am, you know.

"You're being too hard on us. Where's your sense of humor? Sometimes your name is just a punctuation. It doesn't mean anything. We say it . . . just . . . "

In vain?

"Yes. No! Wait a minute!"

Suppose people turned you into a punctuation mark? Besides, it's a bit childish, don't you think, to run around saying God! God! like a kid yanking at his mother's skirt tail: 'Mommie, look! Mama, watch!' . . . By the way, did I ever tell you the story about the little boy who cried 'wolf?'

"Look. I don't know what set you off this morning. Why are you picking on me this way? What's the big deal? What started all this?"

You are the one who called on me, remember?

"So will thousands . . . millions . . . of people today. They don't mean to get you all excited or hurt your feelings. They don't need you; they're just saying your name. That's all."

What do they say when they really do need me?

"God. What is this? Twenty questions?"

No. Just one.

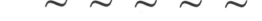

Let's just suppose that Jesus came up to you and personally asked you to sell everything and follow him. What would you do?

U.S. Catholic Magazine conducted a survey asking that question. Here are some of the answers:

"I'd not do such a silly thing."

"Realistically, I don't think he would (ask that)."

"I would, but I would ask him to take care of my wife."

"Perhaps he has already asked and, not recognizing him, I have not followed."

"I can do Christ's work a lot better as I am now than I could if I had nothing."

DOGWOOD DEBS

The dogwoods in my front yard are beginning to look embarrassed. They don't mind being naked in wintertime. In fact, they seem to enjoy it, scratching their bare fingers against the sky like ink pens on a sketch pad.

Dogwoods know how to make the best of a bad situation.

They don't seem to hold a grudge against Old Man Winter, even though he can be rude sometimes — and always leaves them without a stitch to their name.

Dogwoods are creative.

All winter, they dance in the yard, empty-handed and wearing only a smile. They seem perfectly happy in their skimpy winter-black tutus, pirouetting across the lawn in a January wind or doing a stiff-legged fox trot in a February ice storm.

Martha Graham and Alvin Ailey could take a lesson from them, for no dancer could do better when it comes to modern poses and avant-garde contortions than an old dogwood frozen in a *pas de Decembre.*

Now they are tired of winter's game. Impatiently — afraid to get their hopes up — they wait for their new costumes, for a fresh coat of green paint on the dance floor, and for the robins and wrens to take their place in the orchestra pit.

I watched one morning as a skyful of starlings raced by like a gang of noisy children. The dogwoods pretended not to hear because it would only remind them that they were beginning to look silly and were running out of things to keep them amused. Later, a family of chickadees came by to cheer them up, singing a hymn or two in their squeaky soprano voices. The dogwoods clapped politely, but you could tell their hearts were not in it.

Hard as they try, they can't ignore the jonquils and crocuses and hyacinths teasing them underfoot, flaunting gaudy yellows and deep, rich purples — treating the dogwoods like an ugly girl at the prom. Dogwoods are a high-class, well-mannered bunch. They never talk back, but, like all of us, they get their feelings hurt when they are left out or underdressed.

Things have to be pretty bad, though, for a dogwood to start complaining. March is a trying time for them. The weather is so fickle, getting them all worked up with a shower of warm sunlight one day, then letting them down with stinging cold sleet the next.

I heard them talking about this one night as I was coming back from a walk in the neighborhood:

"When are we getting our new outfits?" one whispered to her neighbor. "I can't wait much longer."

"I know how you feel, dear," said another. "It wouldn't be so bad if that forsythia over there would just calm down. It's right tacky the way she sashays back and forth like that . . . so full of herself she almost glows in the dark."

"You're just lucky you don't have a flowering pear right next to you . . ."

And so it went — all up and down the block.

A little later, I found one staring at a patch of Lenten roses, and I know jealousy when I see it. That dogwood was green with envy.

The worst thing of all was what happened in my backyard. A shameless dandelion that somehow got loose and showed up in a bed of ivy underneath an old hemlock took one look at my favorite dogwood and whined in a very loud voice:

"You sure look funny. Didn't your mama teach you how to dress? What are you doing out here stark naked? Don't you know any better than that?"

I hope that hemlock gave it a tongue-lashing when I got out of earshot. Dandelions have no manners.

I know what some of you are saying. You are saying I am crazy. You're saying that anybody who listens to dandelions and talks to trees is crazy as a June bug.

You're right, of course. Everybody goes crazy in the spring, and spring is here. Ready or not. It is official. Today is the first day of spring.

But don't tell the dogwoods. It'll only make them more nervous.

They are doing the best they can.

THE "GOOD" NEWS

From time to time, I get letters from people who feel newspapers in general and I in particular should base every story, every column on what Jesus Christ would say.

Something like that actually happened once.

Jesus Christ — so to speak — "became" the editor of the Topeka Capital on March 13, 1890.

The whole thing started out as a dare between a minister and a newspaper editor. Dr. Charles Sheldon, the 43-year-old pastor of Topeka's Central Congregational Church, looked out one Sunday morning at his bored, dwindling congregation and decided to try something new. Most of his sermons were "from the Bible," as they say: stories about ancient kings, Mideast fishermen, shepherd poets. The same stories week after week, punctuated by hymns so familiar everyone could sing without a book.

He decided to start a series of modern-day, fictional stories that asked the question, "What Would Jesus Do?" Every week, he told a cliff-hanger about a railroad magnate, an heiress, a singer, a college president — all of whom lived messed-up lives until they asked themselves, "What would Jesus do?" and then made their personal or business decisions accordingly.

One of the stories was about a newspaper editor who took a pledge to run his newspaper like Christ would have, which, according to Sheldon, meant no liquor ads, no sensationalism, no gory stories. In Sheldon's Sunday morning story, the man's newspaper flourished, beating out its more worldly competitors, and everybody was the better for it.

Frederick Popenoe, publisher of the Topeka Capital, was in the congregation for that particular sermon and said it would never work that way in real life. He felt so strongly about all this, he challenged Sheldon himself to take on the role of Christ-as-editor for his newspaper for a week and see what happened.

So, between Tuesday, March 13, and Saturday, March 17, 1890, "Jesus" called the shots. Society news was dropped. Stories of crime, scandals, sex and violence were played down. There was no smoking in the newsroom. Ads for alcohol, underwear, entertainment and sporting events were left out. Thousands of advertising dollars from businesses in neighboring Kansas City were turned down because Sheldon felt Christ would want to support small, local shopkeepers.

The Sermon on the Mount ran on the front page. There was not one word printed or one story run that could not be read aloud to the whole family at a church prayer meeting.

Circulation charts exploded. Journalists from all over the world wanted copies. By the end of the five days, the 11,223-circulation Topeka Capital had sold over 362,000 copies to places as far from Kansas as the Boer Republic in South Africa, which was then at war with England.

When Sheldon's editing days were over, he went back to the Central Congregational Church, and circulation returned to normal. Advertisers got back on board, and Sheldon's famous story series became a best-seller, published under the title, "In His

Steps," which was eventually translated into 45 languages and has sold over eight million copies at last count.

The New York Herald ran this assessment of the experiment: "A careful study . . . shows an entire absence of important news of the day. Not a line about bubonic plague at San Francisco, the dreadful tenement house fire at Newark, N.J., the wounding of eight American soldiers in the Philippines, the advance of (General) Roberts on the Orange Free State, the death of the Italian boxer Guydo . . . An article on the first page closes with the remarkable sentence, 'In the Name of Jesus Christ, the Carpenter, the liquor traffic ought to die.' "

So, who won the bet? Was the community better off?

But most of all — who is to decide whether all the decisions and comments came from Jesus Christ?

Or Jesus Sheldon?

~ ~ ~ ~ ~

Does Billy Graham ever cuss? Even on the golf course?

He was asked that once after a bad round, so the story goes, and his answer was what you would expect — plus a twist of characteristic humor:

"No, I don't cuss," he said. " . . . but when I spit, it kills the grass!"

HIGH HOPES

S ome 2,000 years ago, the psalmist
David said that when he needed a
new lease on life, he thought about
the mountains. *I will lift up my eyes
unto the hills . . .*

Odd when you think about it. This poem
was written by a teenage boy who lived in the
desert. Anybody who lives close to the
mountains knows that God's truth is in them.
When we need a dose of Mother Nature's
cure-all, a booster shot against the ills of rut
and routine, we just lift our eyes and there
they are: the mountains.

We can be breathing gas fumes on a city
street, and, if the sun is right, we see them
over yonder, and for a moment nothing else
matters.

We can be dodging death at 60 mph on
the interstate, a million errands half done,
and suddenly there they are, clear as a dream

breaking on the edge of sleep.

And if an eyeful is not enough, we can shove "oughts" and "other plans" under the carpet, throw in a toothbrush and a warm coat, and take to the hills for a transfusion.

No matter if it is cold and nothing is in bloom. No matter that it just snowed. No matter if we really should be doing our taxes. So this past weekend, a friend and I put on our grungies, our serious boots, saddled up the Blazer . . . and took to the hills.

"Awww, I wouldn't try it," the gal in the Stop 'n Go says when we ask about the Deals Gap Road to Fontana. Just what we want to hear. That means the road will be ours. And it is. Riding the dips and curves, the car rocks like a cradle, back and forth, back and forth. The only folks we see are a few early robins, already fat though it's not yet spring; a dozen or so cardinals in their show-off red coats and sassy jester caps; and a jabbering of juncos every time we turn off the road to take a picture or simply pay our respects.

Icicles hang like diamond-studded stalactites alongside the road. Winter clouds push up an opal range of make-believe mountains; an emerald fog of newborn evergreens hovers close to the forest floor.

Winter trees look like macrame, warped and raveled threads stretched on a loom, each a different shade of gray or brown. In spring and summer, you don't notice the color of bark. The green drowns it out, makes it seem insignificant, but it is beautiful: some the color of dove feathers; some like new oyster pearls; some a special blend of hot chocolates.

We stand awhile and listen to the river, a cold green slab telling its story of time in all its tenses. I think about the animals we cannot see, furrowed and burrowed and watching us with sleepy winter eyes. I think about the Native Americans who first took notice and care of this world, then left behind their names: Santeetlah, Cheoah, Wauchecha, Tsali. None of them come in person to check on the two of us, though a red-tailed hawk does fly over with something on his mind as we sit eating a picnic lunch along the Nantahala.

We park in a foot of snow, zip our coats and turn up our collars for a hike through the Joyce Kilmer Memorial Forest. We hear only the crunch of our own footsteps, the drip, drip of snow as it slides down bare fingers of pines and birch.

It's hard to tell the difference, sometimes, between what is dead and what is merely dormant, and we are too often fooled about such things in life. The woods in winter bare secrets told no other place on earth. In just a matter of weeks, these woods will explode, though to judge them from the outside, in the throes of a late spring snow, you'd shrug that idea off as wishful thinking.

I will lift up mine eyes unto the hills . . .

If I didn't know better, I might wonder if, when the psalmist wrote these words, he was sitting on a stone wall beside a busy mountain stream, wearing his warmest mittens and eating Wheat Thins and green grapes.

~   ~   ~   ~   ~

"Americans," Norman Vincent Peale once said, "are so tense and keyed up, it is impossible even to put them to sleep with a sermon."

VI. A BUFFET
OF HOLIDAYS

The hardest job at a newspaper is what copy editors do. They are the never-sleeping sleuths who traipse through story after story looking for misspellings, grammar no-no's, style offenses and all the other dumb mistakes we writers make. I keep them real busy.

Maybe the second hardest job, as far as I am concerned, is thinking up some new column approach to special holidays after, say, fifteen or so years. How many Halloween angles can you come up with? What is there left to say about Santa? Easter eggs? Can you say what needs to be said every Memorial Day without feeling like a broken record? If you get tired of eating the same ol' turkey each Thanksgiving, try writing about it.

At least I'm not the poor copy editor who has to read it over and over, year in and year out.

RESOLVING (AGAIN)

What will we see, and who will we be in the New Year?

No one really knows, of course. Tea leaves, statistics, trends — it's all a guessing game. As we tack the new calendar on the wall, with its 365 blank squares, the best we can do is to recheck our resolutions and wishes for the days ahead.

Here are some of mine.

I resolve (again) to exercise more, eat less and control my temper.

To pay cash.

To look people in the face when I talk.

To laugh at myself, think things through.

To live my intentions, speak my convictions.

To pick my fights carefully.

To write letters like in the olden days, so

189

someday my children's children's children can analyze my
handwriting and hear a voice they never heard ear-to-ear.

To cook turnips and bread pudding for my husband because
he likes them, and to try and forget about the fact that one stinks
up the house and the other tastes like warm vanilla ooze.

Not only to smell more roses, but to help plant them. Also
yellow tulips. Maybe even occasionally to rake leaves.

Not to let a single houseplant die of thirst.

I promise to bug out of my grown children's lives even though
I am full of wise, wonderful, expert, free, ever-ready advice that
could make them perfect and happy forever and ever.

I will listen more than I talk.

Control my greed in book stores and record shops.

Not covet my neighbor's hair.

Not give almond croissants, yeast rolls and anything coconut
more power than they deserve.

I promise to speak up when I hear jokes that aren't really
funny.

I will be more interested in truth than facts.

What do I wish for in the New Year?

I wish places like Somalia and Bosnia needed Weight
Watchers and freezer bags for leftovers.

That Madonna's book and Rush Limbaugh's program couldn't
draw a crowd.

That people would stop ridiculing and terrorizing people
because of who they love in the privacy of their own lives.

That we would all listen to the words we say in church and try
harder to live what they mean. And let God be the judge of who is
doing it better.

I wish little children already born into this world had
advocates as energetic and resourceful as those who might be born.

For all of us to remember that people on the outside of our
circles, those who are the targets of our insults and our prejudices,
all have names, a right to be different and the image of the same
God on their DNA.

That nobody can think of a single good reason to kill a whale,
buy an assault weapon, have a baby unless they can love and take
care of it, start smoking, throw trash on the highway or take more
than their share of anything.

LONG LOST LOVE

Maybe in the long run, love never faileth — but it sure can backfireth. All of us have memories of a painful Valentine massacre somewhere along the line.

The first time my heart made its maiden voyage into the world of True Love, it got smashed to pieces.

May-September romances seldom work out, but I didn't know that then. He was in the 12th grade. I was in the seventh. It was the year they tore down the old junior high school to build a new one, and grades 7-12 crowded into one school on two shifts.

I thanked my lucky stars that he and I ended up on the same shift. Later, if I could've gotten my hands on Cupid, I would have stuck him in the backside with his sharpest arrow.

Because, by the second day of school, I was in love.

His locker was across the hall from mine. He had very white teeth and a Johnny Ray hairdo. His name was Mac.

After months of staring at him through the slits in my locker door, I finally lost my mind. Maybe I ate too many cinnamon red hots or spent too much time listening to the Hit Parade — but that Valentine's Day, I skipped required assembly and left a love letter in Mac's locker.

The only smart thing I did was to sign it "Tiffany."

Tiffany was just one of hundreds of names I wished my parents has used instead of Ina. To me it sounded like the name of a beautiful princess. This was years before Barbie dolls and soap opera names became popular, and there were no Tiffanys in the whole school. I checked.

In those days, people were named after relatives, and as far as I knew nobody else in the whole world had any relatives named Ina. Whatever possessed my parents to give me such a name? It sounded like the name of somebody's pet iguana.

This was the first love letter I ever wrote anybody. All I had to go on was listening to Pat Boone croon about writing "Love Letters in the Sand" and somebody else equally as sappy singing "P.S. I Love You." I did not have beginner's luck.

I told him he was wonderful, which turned out to be a big lie.

Then I really unzipped my heart.

Mac had a certain look about him. His eyes stayed at half mast most of the time. Bedroom eyes, someone at the pajama parties had called them. It drove us seventh-graders crazy.

It is really hard for me to believe I was ever so stupid, but this is — as I told you — a story of TRUE love, emphasis on the true and not "love." Mac's eyes were not his fault.

In my letter I told Mac that a friend of a friend had told me about how he'd lost one of his eyes in that awful car wreck (this was the story making the rounds at the seventh-grade girls' lunch table), that I knew about his GLASS EYE, but I thought it looked real even though sometimes it watered and turned red when he got tired, but that certainly didn't matter to me.

Back then, not only was my brain small, so was my body. I could stand inside my locker and close the door on myself — which is what I did after assembly when Mac returned to his locker to read my letter.

I watched him as — jacket slung over one shoulder, books balanced on his hips — he ripped open the envelope with his white, white teeth.

In my dreams, he would read and reread it slowly, savoring every word and noticing the neat way the "i's" were dotted with little circles. Then he would put it carefully in the pocket closest to his heart. That's what I would have done if someone had written me a letter like that.

On second thought, I'd have probably had an aneurysm.

If you had been standing in that locker with me, you could have heard my heart snap in two when Mac let out that first shout of laughter. He waved my precious secret in the air and, killing me softly with every whoop and holler, asked if everybody wanted to see something hard to believe.

All that day, his friends called him Cyclops.

Turns out he didn't have a glass eye after all. Just hay fever.

I spent the rest of that day in my locker, blowing my nose on my gym shorts. As soon as I got home, I worked up a cough that by suppertime had my mother worried I might be coming down with something. My temperature turned out to be 103, thanks to the old run-the-thermometer-under-warm-water trick.

Anything to get out of school for the rest of my life.

All that winter and spring, Cyclops (the name stuck) walked the halls with his arms around this girl or that from a harem of cheerleaders, student government presidents and May Court queens. I lived in horror that one day he would have a vision and learn that Tiffany was really the girl who jumped inside her locker every time he rounded the corner.

The gods were with me on that score. He never knew. My luck got better, and soon I even forgot, but not without learning something: Love not only can warm the cockles of the heart . . . it can burn holes in it.

Whoever decided it was better to have loved and lost than not to have loved at all never fell for an older man with hay fever.

SOMETIMES IT'S BETTER NOT TO ASK

We can't let the first day of April slip by without one foolish story.

Once upon a time — or so it goes — there was a schoolteacher in a small Midwestern town who felt life was passing her by. Every morning, she went to the same school, taught the same subjects, came home to the same house, watched the same TV programs and went to bed at the same time every night.

Life was dull.

She wished she had the nerve to do something different. Something daring.

One day, she read a magazine article about Scotland in National Geographic. She could almost smell the heather, hear the bagpipes. The people seemed to walk off the page right into her heart. She could even imagine the moors calling her by name.

"Aha!" she said to herself. "This is it!"

Well, the long and short of it is that she took a trip to Scotland for the summer. It was all she dreamed it would be. She felt the old kinks in her life iron themselves out among the lochs and thistles. She didn't want to go home.

When she saw a newspaper ad for a schoolteacher in a friendly little town she was visiting, she threw caution to the wind and applied for the job. The minister at the Wayside Chapel — a kind and gentle man with a twinkle in his eyes — said he knew a place she could get a room. He would make the arrangements. So, she went back home to turn in her resignation, settle her affairs and pack.

Then she began to get cold feet.

What sort of place would the minister find for her to live in? Would it be quiet? Would it be clean? What about privacy? In her nightmares, she saw herself sharing a grungy bathroom down the hall with all sorts of riffraff, or having hot water only once a week, by appointment. Or always being afraid someone would walk in on her.

She decided her peace of mind was worth the nerve it would take to write the minister and ask about the bathroom situation.

Only, she couldn't bring herself to use the word "bathroom." Especially to a man of the cloth! Nice ladies didn't use that word. Besides, he wouldn't know what she was talking about. They had another name for it. What was it, now? Water closet. Yes, that was it.

So, she wrote the minister and asked him to describe where she would be living. For example, where was the . . . uh . . . she finally decided on using just the initials.

When the minister got the letter, he was confused.

What could she mean by "W.C."? The only W.C. he could think of was the water closet — but didn't Americans call it the "bathroom"? He decided she must be talking about his beloved Wayside Chapel. How nice of her to ask.

So, with enthusiasm, he wrote back this letter:

"The W.C. is located in the center of town, right on the Town Square. Since it is the only one within 50 miles, it is where people gather to catch up on the news, to swap recipes, to leave their children while they shop . . . as well as to say their prayers and sing hymns.

"On Sundays, people from all around come for the day and bring their lunch. Those who live close by come regularly, but in bad weather, some of the farmers and sheep herders can't go for months at a time.

"Recently, we put in beautiful windows, and at present we are raising money for a new organ. The music in the W.C. is some of the most beautiful you will ever hear. Do you like to sing? We hope so. Perhaps you would like to read for us sometimes in the W.C.

"Some of the ladies have agreed to needlepoint cushions with everyone's family crest.

"I'm sure you will feel right at home in our little W.C., and soon everyone will be looking for you in your special place. You know how people are about always wanting to sit in the same place. Maybe you will meet some nice young man next to you.

"We hope the W.C. is one of the first places you will want to go to when you arrive in town. In fact, we'll pin a ribbon on you at your first visit, so everyone will come over and speak . . ."

The last I heard, poor thing, she was still watching TV in the same old den.

JESUS IN THE GARDEN

This isn't about bunnies or egg hunts, and it didn't happen at Easter, but it's a Holy Week story just the same. It's about a little girl I'll call Mandy, because long ago when all this happened, Mandy was the name of her favorite doll — the same doll now packed away in the attic, waiting to be a grand-doll-baby.

When Mandy was 4 years old, she had a little red plastic car. Every morning, she put her dolls in the seat beside her and drove up and down the driveway — talking to herself and hushing up her children when they got out of hand, as all mothers do.

One of her rituals was to mail a pretend letter or two at her pretend post office — which was a place on the wall at the end of the driveway where somebody's bumper had knocked out two bricks.

Mandy's father was a gardener, and every spring he'd start hauling in straw and transplanting monkey grass and come home from the hardware store with baby impatiens and sweet William.

That Christmas, his mother-in-law broke from tradition and didn't send him the usual tie or red V-neck. She gave him a statue of St. Francis of Assisi for his garden.

By Christmas night, the beautiful stone statue of St. Francis was carefully placed under the plum tree in a bed of wintering ivy. It was a perfect spot because it hid the unsightly chink in the brick wall — the one that Mandy had turned into a post office.

The next morning, Mandy set out on her errands in the little red car.

And that's when she found Jesus.

Who else could it be? It was, after all, the day after Christmas. She'd never heard of St. Francis, but she knew about Jesus — and there he was, smiling at her and holding a little bird in his hands. She felt like she had made a wonderful, important discovery. God must have put him there just for her.

She didn't tell anyone and nobody mentioned the fact that Jesus was standing in the ivy right there in their backyard, so Mandy figured he had meant it to be their little secret. Every day she went to see Jesus in the garden, talking to him and singing the songs she learned in Sunday school. Once, when she was sent to her room for sassing her mother, Mandy stood at the window and looked out at Jesus, and it made her feel better in a mysterious way.

When spring came that year, Mandy's daddy decided one Saturday morning that St. Francis would look better standing in the gerber daisies. He could plant an azalea in front of Mandy's post office.

As he picked up the statue, it slipped through his fingers, and St. Francis fell against the wall. It knocked a hole in his shoulder and sliced off part of his face. Mandy's father carefully gathered up the pieces and put the statue in the tool shed, making a mental note to get some glue from the hardware store to patch it up.

Just before supper, Mandy drove over to say good night to Jesus.

But he wasn't there.

She looked everywhere. He had simply vanished. Was God

mad at her? Was it because she had scribbled "I hate Mom" on the
back of the door in red crayon?

Mandy picked at her supper that night. She said her prayers
over and over, blessing everyone she knew — especially her
mother. Why had Jesus paid her a special visit and then
disappeared into thin air, like it had all been a dream or a game of
let's pretend?

The next morning when Mandy went to get her little red car
out of the tool shed, what she found broke her heart. It was Jesus,
lying on his side. His face looked grotesque, like something from a
horror movie. By the time she got to the kitchen, Mandy was
crying so hard she developed hiccups, and her mother could hardly
understand what she was saying.

Something about Jesus in the tool shed.

It took a long time to sort things out. Theology and catechisms
cover a lot of territory, and library shelves are full of books on child
rearing that anticipate just about everything. But nowhere can you
find exactly what to say to a 4-year-old who thinks her daddy
killed Jesus and put him in the tool shed.

That was a long time ago. "Mandy" is now grown.

But every spring, when St. Francis gets moved to a better spot
in the garden — this year, he's standing in the Lenten roses —
Mandy's mother and father think about that day and how upset
Mandy had been. They remember how hard it was to explain why
Jesus didn't live inside a cement statue. How he doesn't have to
depend on us to glue him back together.

And that even when you write ugly words on the back of the
door or drop something precious and it breaks — even when
something seems dead — it's not the end of the world.

TIME OUT
FOR PEACE

Memorial Day. Time to remember. Most of us won't think too much today about bombs bursting and body bags.

Most of us will sleep late, clean the gutters, play with the kids.

Memorial Day originated when Southern women — widows, mothers, sisters, daughters, grandmothers — decided to organize wreath-layings on their Confederate dead.

Maybe it's time for women to organize again. To protest.

To go to war on war.

To shout, carry placards, stage sit-ins.

To say, "No more."

No longer will we kiss our sons and daughters good-bye, pack their toothbrushes and send them off to places we cannot pronounce. Or even those we can.

Maybe it's time we leave our knitting, our nests, our offices, our tenements, our kitchens, our boardrooms, our pews, our tennis courts, our rice paddies and say — all together now — "No more!"

Women find no fascination in war.

You'd have a hard time getting the mothers of the world to push the button, to pull the plug.

They'd never be ready to aim, then fire. Not because they can't understand ideologies and politics, old wounds and old sayings, but because there is bound to be a better answer.

Sooner or later we all get our wars and the reasons for them mixed up.

What was the fighting about?

It only gets sorted out on history tests, and even then the answers have to be memorized. It simply does not make sense to kill each other's children. Grown or otherwise.

Ask any mother. She'd agree. The lullabies in any language are the same.

If we could somehow see a snapshot of the "child" in our gun sights, we'd have no stomach to kill him.

Maybe when things go wrong, instead of briefings and strategies and maps with pins in them, we should swap family stories and photos.

Would it work?

Maybe. We've tried everything else.

Maybe women need to organize once more a memorial for their dead, this time by refusing to go to war ever again.

Refusing to believe that the best she can do after war is over is to lay a wreath and, while it is going on, to bandage her bleeding soul and breaking heart with prayer.

"Please, dear God, bring him home. Spare him." Mothers on all sides are praying the same prayer.

So whose baby should it be in the body bag?

Why should — can — anybody's God choose which of his children to wipe out, anymore than we could. Or would.

Whose baby should it be?

Nobody's. Ask any mother. She'll tell you, and she won't even have to stop to consider what flag was stitched to the uniform.

So maybe the mothers of the world need to call a meeting. Take, say, the money we spend in one day getting ready for war and offer a plane ticket to a delegation of mothers from all over the world.

A "Show and Tell" for peace.

First, they'd show pictures of their children:

Red and yellow, black and white. Precious in anybody's sight.

Then, tell the world, "No more war."

Would it work? Sillier pipe dreams have been laughed at and tossed out.

The world did turn out to be round.

We have been to the moon.

It's at least worth a thought today as we plant our gardens and watch our kids play.

Think about it as taps blows at Arlington on the 6 o'clock news. And, when the cameras pan across the military cemeteries of America for their Memorial Day feature, imagine each grave as a kind of cradle, where some mother's child is laid, as he or she once was, side by side with others.

In a nursery.

Summer, n: 1."*The season when kids slam the doors they've left open all winter.*" — *Dave Garroway.* 2. "*The time of year when the highway authorities close the regular roads and open up the detours.*" — *Herbert Victor Prochnow.* 3. "*The time of year when all the women who aren't at the beach get undressed anyway and go to the supermarket.*" — *Anonymous.*

Summertime, n: 1. *when parents pack off their troubles to an old Indian camp and smile, smile, smile.*

TAKING STOCK, SEEKING FORGIVENESS

Yom Kippur is the holiest day in the Jewish calendar.

I apologize ahead of time to any person who finds misunderstanding or oversimplification of what this holy day means to them. It would certainly be unreasonable to think someone who was not part of my own Christian/ Presbyterian background could best explain, say, Maundy Thursday or John Calvin. My husband remembers being in a Moscow museum one summer when he was on a student exchange to the Soviet Union. In explaining a Russian icon entitled "The Holy Family," the guide pointed to Mary and said, "This is God's . . . uh . . . mistress."

Was he making fun or being intentionally offensive? Of course not.

I suppose that's why religious wars (and discussions) are often the bloodiest.

Misunderstandings easily turn to judgments that breed anger.

Yom Kippur slips by most years with my hardly noticing, which to a Jew is as hard to deal with as my thinking Easter might be just another day. But, no matter our own religious convictions, it would do us all good to take stock and seek forgiveness today.

That, as I understand it, is at the core of Yom Kippur.

Jewish tradition says that for the past 10 days God has been studying a book that records everyone's deeds during the past year. This 10th day of their New Year — called Yom (Hebrew word for "day") Kippur (meaning "atonement") — is a time to pray from sunup to sundown for God to have mercy on them for their sins and to look favorably on them in the days to come.

In ancient times, animal sacrifices were offered on Yom Kippur, as was the custom in most early religious and mystic rituals. Biblical instructions for Yom Kippur bind not only Jews, but all of us whose religious roots are in the Old Testament, to this holy day. The specifics on how it is to be observed are recorded in detail in several passages. For instance, here are our instructions from portions of Leviticus 16:

"This shall become a rule binding on you for all time. On the tenth day of the seventh month you shall mortify yourselves; you shall do no work, whether native Israelite or alien settler, because on this day expiation shall be made on your behalf to cleanse you, and to make you clean before the Lord from all your sins. The priest shall burn the fat of the sin offering upon the altar . . ."

There have, of course, been modifications of these observances, just as we have changed some of the "rules" of New Testament worship, such as covered heads, common treasuries, the place and style of music and liturgy.

On Yom Kippur, Jews gather in their synagogues and temples to seek forgiveness from God and others in prayer and corporate worship. The more primitive aspects of the instructions have been, in practice, "edited out" — for lack of a better word, I admit — with no loss to its original and sacred meaning.

Besides the spiritual implications of Yom Kippur for all people of faith, this holy day has left its mark in the English language.

The word "scapegoat" gets its meaning from the second of two goat offerings made in ancient times on this "Day of Atonement." The first goat was an offering to Yahweh. The second, called the scapegoat, was to Azazel, the spirit of evil.

When time came for the priest to raise this goat to be sacrificed, he recited and confessed the sins of the people. Then, he let the goat loose, allowing it to scamper off into the wilderness unharmed.

This became the moment of forgiveness.

Today, a person who is blamed, as the goat was, for something that is the fault of somebody else is called a scapegoat. The symbolism of that act is lived out every day in a thousand ways.

No matter who we are or what we do or do not believe, you and I are let off the hook more times than we deserve.

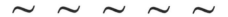

October is a misnomer. Octo means "eight" in Latin, and when the Roman calendar — predecessor of the Gregorian calendar we use today — was drawn up, October was the eighth month, not the 10th. So, if you want to get technical, today is the first day of December. Decem is ten. Of course that messes up December, the former 10th month. How about Xober and Twelvember?

THANKSGIVING IN PROPER PERSPECTIVE

There's a Thanksgiving feast being served up, free of charge, over in the Smokies at Porters Flat. Actually, this kind of feast has more in common with what was served our forefathers in New England (or Virginia, depending on which "First Thanksgiving" story you pick) than the kind of celebrating we do in our cozy dens and dining rooms.

The first Pilgrims didn't even have turkey. They ate eel. They didn't play football, either. Or watch Charlie Brown specials. They certainly didn't shop till they dropped, bagging bargains at the sales.

They did, however, have the same feast for their eyes we have spread around us in these mountains.

The bountiful harvest of autumn's last gasp.

It is the season most like life as we know

it this side of the river. The seasons of our days play out the good-news-bad-news forecast of late November. Life is a late fall landscape. Sooner or later we learn from experience that green pastures are most beautiful when they stand under bare mountains. That stars shine clearest in a cold sky. That the sun is its most golden when the earth tilts and the shadows fall.

In real life, blessings are mixed in with losses.

Since moving to East Tennessee, late fall has become one of my favorite times of year. For me, a pilgrimage to places like Porters Flat is the best way to celebrate the Thanksgiving season. It is a banquet for the soul, mind, heart.

Porters Creek trail follows the river, weaving its way along a magic carpet of leaves under a stained-glass ceiling of hemlock, red maple, blue sky and beams of laser sunlight. An old cemetery thrives under a shroud of brambles and fallen trees, up a little hill to the right. Most of the graves are children's graves from the early 1900s. Stop to read the names, the dates. And count your blessings. Things not only could be worse . . . back in those days, they were:

Little Rosalia, whose light flickered only a day. Only one among four, five, six tiny markers in the same family plot, each with dates and verses hand-carved in mossy stones.

Dates and verses carved, no doubt, in the weathered faces and hearts of those who watched and waited until the watching and waiting were over.

Old men sleeping next to mothers who died hardly out of their teens, probably in childbirth. Cousins from three generations sharing the same piece of earth.

Standing there, listening to voices from my own past and hearing the rush of water over rocks in a nearby creek, the words to an old hymn seem to hang in the air: *Time like an ever rolling stream bears all its sons away* . . . How true.

The next line, though certainly poetic, bothers me.

They fly forgotten as the dream breaks at the opening day.

Maybe we can keep that from happening to the people we love if we take time to remember and give thanks . . . for the living as well as those whose names are carved on gravestones in our family cemeteries.

Celebrating our memories, awakened so naturally by the

sights and sensations of this season's silent exit, should be the main course in our Thanksgiving banquet. When I need to be reminded of that, places like Porters Flat put it all in perspective.

It's the sowing and tilling of memories, the harvesting and milling of family relationships that, ultimately, fill our barns with blessings enough to carry us through all the seasons of life.

WHEN LOVE GOES DINGDONG

It wasn't so bad the first day.

The doorbell rang, and there he was, holding a little bush with a bird sitting in it.

"It's a partridge," he said, "in a pear tree."

"Awwww," I grinned. "Isn't he cute? And you know how I like pears. Gee, thanks."

Wasn't that nice? Such an unusual gift. Not the kind of thing you get in a catalog or at the drugstore at the last minute. He's a love.

The second day I was out in the backyard planting my tree, and the doorbell rang again. There he stood with another partridge in another pear tree and two live things on his head.

"Oh, dear," I said. "You shouldn't have."

"This is Jack and this is Suzy," he said. "They are turtledoves."

How can you get mad with something as romantic as that? Besides I love pears. He's such a love. Truly.

When the doorbell rang on the third day, I began to get a little nervous. This time he had three hens scratching around in my azaleas, another tree and two more turtledoves cooing away on top of his head.

"Hon," I said, "I really appreciate the thought, but . . . ."

"They're French," he said.

"What?"

"The hens. They are French. Very expensive. Very tasty. Delicious on toast points with hollandaise."

Well. We all have our little peculiarities. If he likes to give weird gifts, who am I to judge?

On the fourth day, I was in the kitchen putting up who knows how many pecks of pickled pears when there was a knock at the door.

Oh, Lord. Would you believe four new birds? Three more French chickens? Another pair of doves? Plus a fourth dadgum partridge in a tree?

"Sweetheart, could we have a little talk?" I said. "What's with all the birds? Is there a message I'm not getting? Just tell me. I give up."

"Know what a cally bird is?" he asked. "It's a blackbird. Betcha didn't know that, huh? Makes a delicious pie. Mix up four and 20 of these little babies, a little sugar, bake at 350 for about an hour and when the pie is opened, guess what?"

"What?"

"They sing!"

You think you know someone when you're in love, but maybe mother was right. Exactly how many marbles does he have? Is that a full deck he is holding? On the other hand, maybe it's not so bad. Maybe he just has this need to . . . well . . . to bring birds, or something.

By the fifth day, I was a wreck. I had just finished baking crepe Suzettes and coq Saint-Jacques and was on the phone talking with the Service Master people about an estimate on dove droppings.

Then, dingdong.

I knew it wasn't one of the neighbors. We were no longer

speaking. They'd left threatening notes, asking who did I think I was, Dr. Doolittle? I almost threw up when I saw him there with two more pigeons on his head, another flock of birds and hens, and you guessed it! A partridge and a pear tree.

"THIS HAS GOT TO STOP," I shouted. "THIS IS THE SEASON FOR LOVE AND JOY AND PEACE. YOU ARE NUTS, DO YOU KNOW THAT? A REAL, TRUE, LIVE BIRDBRAIN."

But then he took out this little box and inside were . . . fi-hive go-ooold rings. Real gold. One for every other finger. Of course, I'd have to take them off to gather eggs and work in the orchard — but next to pears, I really love rings.

So, what's a little silliness between two people crazy in love? After all, life is serious enough as it is. We kissed and made up. He's a love. The next day, I was pricing 800 feet of chicken wire and was just going out to get my rings sized when the doorbell rang. No. It couldn't be. It just couldn't be.

But it was.

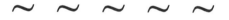

"It is my heart-warm and world-embracing Christmas hope and aspiration that all of us, the high, the low, the rich, the poor, the admired, the despised, the loved, the hated, the civilized, the savage (every man and brother of us all throughout the whole earth), may eventually be gathered together in a heaven of everlasting rest and peace and bliss, except the inventor of the telephone."
— *Mark Twain*

WITH APOLOGIES TO CLEMENT MOORE

T is the week before Christmas, and all through the house, everybody is stirring. There's so much noise and confusion that any mouse with half a brain has packed up and moved out.

The stockings aren't hung yet because nobody can find them. They were supposed to be wrapped around the lights, but every box in the attic has been plowed through so many times it looks like there's been a train wreck up there.

Mama says Santa made off with them, darn his time. Dad says Santa is getting senile, darn hers.

A piece of the manger scene is also missing. One king was killed off sometime during the summer, up there in the attic.

How about a new trend: "We two kings from Orient are . . . "

The Bible doesn't say exactly how many there were, anyway.

The moon isn't on the crest of the new-fallen snow. At least not in our backyard. It's ricocheting off dark plastic forms of garbage bags too numerous to fit in the cans. Where does it all come from?

Where does it all go?

But Clement Moore got one thing right.

Santa's belly is so stuffed with lemon squares and cookie dough she doesn't need any pillows to make it shake like a bowl full of jelly. Even when she isn't laughing.

'Tis the week before Christmas, and no children I know anything about are nestled all snug in their beds. They're too busy driving Mom crazy with the school band program, the church pageant and a pajama party.

All the same night.

Then there is Christmas music. It's hard to keep your wits about you when you have an 8-year-old who has just learned to play "Deck the Halls" on the piano. Sort of. After about the 46th verse — before lunch — those fa-la-la-las start hammering on your sinuses.

What Mama can take a long winter's nap this time of year? What father can settle his brain? It's a challenge just to stay sane.

'Tis the week before Christmas, and nobody at our house has once mentioned sugarplums. Sugarplums — whatever they are — are a thing of the past. Kids today want Nerf Archery Sets which are nowhere to be found in the civilized world. The visions dancing in their heads are of Super Nintendo, designer jeans — even family ski trips that not only don't fit into Santa's pack, but cost more than it used to cost him to feed, house and entertain all his elves, all winter long.

It certainly is hard to give a wink of the eye and a nod of the head and tell the children they have nothing to dread when — the week before Christmas — the postman brings the credit card bills, the tax forms and two life insurance premium notices all in the same mail. When ol' Santa comes home to that, his eyes don't twinkle a bit. No, siree. His hands start to tremble, and his eyebrows meet and he mumbles, "Who do they think I am, J. Paul Getty?"

'Tis the week before Christmas, and, no, Virginia dear, there really aren't such things as reindeer. The Dasher or Comet sitting out back with the iffy front tire and dirty windshield eats gas, not grass. Its driver isn't all that lively and quick, either. In fact, she's exhausted.

"Mom, I got play practice" . . . "Mom! Take me to the mall."

So, it's dash away, dash away, dash away, all. Back and forth. Back and forth. The dog eats 12 candy canes and a tin of fudge. To the vet's. A 17-year-old spills soup on his only dress pants. To the cleaner's. Sixteen new movies hit town the day school is out. To the movies. There's no Scotch tape. To the drug store.

'Tis the week before Christmas and all through the house are secrets and loud music, lists and no money. The kitchen floor is gritty with sugar, and the kids have rattled the presents under the tree so many times the tags are falling off.

There are traffic jams and post office lines, a turkey to stuff, fresh coconut to grate, bills to pay, phones ringing off the wall, no place to sit in the den and never any hot water when it's your turn in the shower.

'Tis the week before Christmas, and I don't feel like an elf. But what do I do?

Laugh in spite of myself.

THE FINAL VERSE

One Christmas — I guess I was about 8 or 9 — my father took me with him on a visit to a nursing home. He was a Presbyterian minister and would often, as he put it, "pay a call" on shut-ins in the congregation.

Lots of times he took one of us along, especially around Christmas. Usually when he went to the critical care unit of a nursing home, we waited in the car; but, for some reason this particular Christmas, I tagged along.

As we opened the heavy swinging doors that separated the sick from the well, I entered a world unlike anything I had known, and I was more frightened than I remember ever being before and maybe even since.

Going to visit older people had always been something I looked forward to. I got "oooed" and "ahhed" over, and, when talk

shifted from me to something else, I most times had a candy cane
to lick or a Whitman Sampler to keep me busy.

I liked the way my father had of making people laugh, and I
felt important belonging to him. But this was different. These
people did not look like people at all. They looked like bodies left
behind after the people who lived in them had gone somewhere. I
did not understand or want any part of what I saw and felt.

My father went to each bed, speaking gently to the patients,
most of whom said nothing but lay like grown-up rag dolls in the
half darkness.

There were pictures on the dresser: A lady in a pretty hat
laughing at a baby on her hip; a kind-looking man in a business
suit almost winking into the camera. I knew what name tags were.
These must have been face tags, reminding nurses and doctors and
strangers like me that these lost, forgotten people were once real.

Several wept silently. Most slept. A few looked at me and said
nothing. Others looked through me, saying things I could not
understand. One man thought my daddy was his daddy, and,
coming alive at the recognition, called out in a little boy voice that
did not match his face, "Please, take me home."

A group of Christmas carolers came through the hall, and, as
they got closer, I recognized what they were singing. It was "Joy to
the World."

How cruel, I thought.

How inappropriate.

Just then, I heard a voice from across the hall call out, "Little
girl? Little girl? Come here."

I'd have never budged, except that my father took me by the
shoulder and led the way.

"How old are you?" the voice wanted to know. I couldn't
remember.

"Would you sing that song to me?"

. . . and I wouldn't have if my father hadn't gotten me started.

And hea-ven and hea-ven and na-ture sing.

"Do you know the last verse?" the voice said.

"No, ma'am," I whispered.

"Promise me something, my dear." she said. "Learn it. It's the
best verse of all."

We rode home in silence, my father and I. When we pulled up

in the driveway and he turned off the car engine, neither of us got out.

"Why?" I asked. "I don't understand how God can let these people be like that."

It was a perfect time for a sermon. I was hanging on for some passage of Scripture, some simple sentence to memorize that would answer all such questions forever and ever.

Instead, my father said, "I don't know."

He waited for that to sink in and then went on. "But she is right. The last verse of 'Joy to the World' promises us that even when we are not who we are, even when it looks like we have been left behind or feel alone — we can depend on the mystery of God's love."

The older I get, the more I think about those words in the last verse and all the other "wonders of love" we discover in this life.

Both of those voices from that night have long since been silenced, but their words ring in my ears as I celebrate Christmas.

And wonder still.

VII. CRAZY PEOPLE AND OTHER SOUTHERN PHENOMENA

I have this ongoing argument with my Yankee friends. They say we Southerners are hung up on the subject of our roots, our point of view, our traditions.

"Y'all aren't all that special," they say. Only they don't say "y'all." And they don't know what the heck they are talking about. Of course there is something extra special about the South. We have more sense of place than any other part of the country.

In fact, we have more sense of place than any other sense. We're nuts on the subject.

Which proves my point.

THE SANDS OF TIME

It's deja vu all over again.

A thousand trips I've taken over these dunes, down to the water. Most of them, or so it seems, with a baby on my hip and one or two trudging alongside.

Rubber rafts hooked through my arm, towels draped over my shoulders, sun oil and toys bouncing along in a canvas papoose. Chairs, coolers, umbrellas, snacks . . .

I hit the beach like a Parris Island Marine on maneuvers.

But this summer was different.

One daughter is on a month's hiking trip in Wyoming. I see her, in my mind's eye, weighing less than the backpack she is now carrying . . . struggling up the baby dunes in tiny flip-flops and huge Barbie sunglasses.

Another "child" is somewhere between New Mexico and Houston, in her own car, going back to her own house, her own class of

221

fourth-graders next week.

I imagine her paddling along behind me, too. I remember how she'd never allow anyone to carry her at the scary end of the pier, its wide-set boards just about big enough to swallow a 3-year-old whole. She was scared, but she wanted to do it her own self.

The years don't seem that far away as I stand atop the dunes and watch the waves play along the beaches of all my memories.

Our son, George, is joining us for the weekend, up from Charleston, where he just finished college and is afloat in the real world, determined to earn enough money for graduate school.

It's a 500-mile trip for us, from Knoxville to Wrightsville Beach, N.C., back to this old house where we've come for vacations every summer since time began for us as a family.

And every summer of my own childhood was spent here.

On the way down from the Knoxville mountains, the rain hits the windshield hard as marbles, and, when it stops, a thick heat lies across I-40 like hot compresses.

But Saturday on the beach is wonderful. We do all our beach things.

Carswell beats us in a game of Russian Bank.

George beats us in a game of Sniglet.

I beat them out of fixing ANY meals.

Saturday afternoon, while Carswell sleeps in the hammock and the sky spits rain, George and I go to Redix — the beach-junk, T-shirt, postcard capital of the world. I used to take the kids there on rainy afternoons at least once during our two weeks at Wrightsville, giving them $3 to spend on whatever. It kept them busy for hours.

For old time's sake, George and I give each other $3 and head straight for the toys.

The old favorites are still there: Plastic snakes. Matchbox cars. Paint-by-number things. Silly Putty. Slinkeys. Sand sculpture tools. Magic sets. Comic books.

Finally, he decides on blow bubbles and Snap 'n Pops. I get two water guns and a jacks set.

We spend the afternoon blowing bubbles off the porch and shooting them with water guns. Then, he beats me in jacks. I blame it on arthritis, but he knows better. I've NEVER gotten past "threesies." Maybe there's a bone missing in my hand.

We throw Snap 'n Pops to wake Carswell in time to take us out for Italian food.

It is great swimming in the ocean at sunset. We ride the surf until our knees are skinned up. The waves are the biggest I have seen in recent memory. When you dive under, they zoom over like muffled jets, stirring up so much foam the water out to the breakers turns into a huge aerial map of the world.

It is too muggy to sleep, so Sunday morning I get up way before light and walk to the inlet and back, then climb up the lifeguard stand to watch the sun come up.

It is magenta.

George and I rock on the porch, talking about life and listening to his music. He says he told his biology professor he simply WOULD NOT cut open a cat, even if it meant he'd fail. They worked out that he would study off someone else's; he ended up getting an A and one less cat bit the dust. He's like that, but it's something he'd probably never have told me except at the beach.

There's something about salt water and sandy thunderstorms that loosens the tongue and washes the soul.

It was always that way with us.

Except this time, it is George who carries *my* stuff over the dunes, down to the edge.

COMMON AS KUDZU

O l' Santa might be a gall-darned Yankee, sledding in each year from as far up north as you can get, but the best presents inside his treasure pack come from Southern writers.

The wet wax-paper weather that sets in after Christmas is the perfect time to curl up with a book and tell each other stories. Nothing drowns out the sound of rain better than opening a new book and hearing that crack of unchartered pages.

Southern writers have something special going for them. I don't exactly know what it is, but it's there. Eudora Welty, Josephine Humphries, William Faulkner, Joyce Carol Thomas, Clyde Edgerton, Flannery O'Connor — they all have it, though style and subject matters differ.

More and more I am convinced: Molly Ivins' sassy political columns, a new T.R.

Pearson novel, and an early Cormac McCarthy book I had not yet read. It's like they came from the same family, despite the fact that their books are planets apart in shape and intent.

Maybe it's something stirred up in grits, something that comes out of the ground and into the lungs from smoking rabbit tobacco. Maybe it's a quark-like chemical emitted from kudzu or backwoods gin.

Whatever it is, all Southern writers have it.

Despite what our magazines would have us believe, Southern living is not just about Mardi Gras and mimosa, Cajun cooking and putting greens. Southern living is telling stories. Southerners use stories to explain everything: our politics, our religion, our roots, our prides and our prejudices.

All people do this, I realize, but Southerners do it with — I don't know — a flair.

Even our lies are true. Even when we exaggerate, we tell it like it is.

Pat Conroy once told me people come up to him all the time and ask how come he knows so many strange people. How come so many of them are in his own family?

His "pat" answer (sorry) is that he just pays attention. There are crazy people everywhere in the South, he says.

In fact, we're all crazy.

If they stand there looking at him like he is, indeed, living, breathing proof of this lopsided opinion, he asks if they are from the South, and if they are he asks "quite seriously," how far back in their own family do they have to go to uncover the oddballs, the secrets, the hushed-up mysteries.

Is he saying that Southerners are more likely to be crazy than, say, someone from New Jersey?

I don't know. But try it.

Ask any Southerner, and he or she can reel off in a heartbeat a list of crazies they have known: holed up behind shutters or talking to themselves during church or elected to the Legislature. Southern families on both sides of the tracks have them sitting on every branch in the family tree.

And these strange, myth-like creatures grow taller or meaner or more eccentric with every story.

By the time we reach the fifth grade, every small-town

Southerner can write a report on "Monsters I Have Known on a First-Name Basis" . . . mysterious neighbors who come out only at night from houses with weeds up to the windowsills; pale women who live with a hundred cats or push empty baby carriages.

Stuffy, strict old-maidish uncles who terrify small children with their laser-beam eyes and a death clutch on manners. Second cousins who can say the whole Pledge of Allegiance during one long burp. The grandfather who refuses to use a turn signal or give in to windshield wipers.

And, of course, there is being sickly, Southern style. Everyone of us has a cousin or neighbor somewhere along the line who took poorly at 32 and devoted her life to getting ready for the Big Exit. Her whole house smelled of cough drops and stale whispers. It was no shock to anyone except herself that she died at 102. Of what? Natural causes. In her sleep.

With, at last, a smile.

~ ~ ~ ~ ~

From Oscar Wilde's "Impressions on America" — written in 1882:

Among the more elderly inhabitants of the South, I found a melancholy tendency to date every event of importance by the late war.

"How beautiful is the moon tonight," I once remarked to a gentleman who was standing next to me.

"Yes," was his reply, "but you should have seen it before the war."

THE GRITTY TRUTH

One thing I've learned in my year and a half in Knoxville is that it is not a 100-percent Dixie-fied city. Some folks around here actually wore blue during the War of Northern Aggression (ha!) and not everyone drinks mint juleps under the magnolias on a warm summer day.

But the real tip-off is that grits is not a staple on every restaurant menu nor does it come automatically on every breakfast order.

I actually got served hash browns the other day.

I hate to make sweeping generalizations, but I think something is missing from Northern mentality when it comes to grits.

Take, for instance, the time my husband and I were eating breakfast at The Homestead in Hot Springs. A bunch of the guests were at one long table. On our right

227

was a man from Boston. A lawyer. A Harvard man, no less. On the left was an insurance salesman from Philadelphia who had one of those million-dollar roundtable pins in his lapel.

They were both very smart.

I knew that because they read The Wall Street Journal and used words like "eclectic" and "infrastructure" before they'd had any coffee. They were savvy fellows, too. Not just brain-smart eggheads. They knew which of the six forks to use and always passed the cream pitcher to you handle first.

Anyway, there we all were at breakfast.

When the waitress came around with the grits, Boston and Philadelphia wanted to know what they were.

My husband is from Georgia, the state where grits were invented, so he told them.

"Grits," he said, trying to be helpful. "You know, Georgia ice cream."

They didn't even smile. They were too busy looking into the bowl, sniffing, poking the spoon around.

Then they both turned up their noses.

"No, thanks."

Now wait just a minute, I thought. Grits don't smell. They don't look funny. But these Yankees treated that bowl of grits like something going through airport security.

"What exactly are grits made of?" asked Harvard. "Is it a seed or what?"

"No, they grow on trees," I said, thinking he was surely joking.

"What kind of tree?" asked Philadelphia.

"A grit tree," my husband piped in.

They didn't bat an eye. Neither did we.

"Really?" one said.

"No kidding?" said the other.

I guess what happened next just goes to show how one lie leads to another.

"Well, yes," said Georgia. "We were just kidding. Actually, a grit is a little animal that lives in South Carolina, Georgia, Mississippi — places like that. It's small . . . white . . . has little red eyes . . ."

Boston and Philadelphia just kept chewing their rye toast.

"We have a few grits in Georgia," my husband went on, in his best Barney Fife-Uncle Remus voice. ". . . but the true grit comes from around Charleston and up towards Richmond."

At this point, the waitress appeared with what Boston and Philadelphia had chosen of their own free will off the menu. It looked like something you'd find on the floor in a Friday the Thirteenth movie. Lox, they called it.

And it did smell.

". . . the salt marsh Indians of the Low Country," continued my husband, trying to breathe through his mouth to avoid lox fumes, "used the grit's paw as a symbol of divine protection. In special ceremonial rites, as soon as it was weaned from its mother, every Southern native American's son or daughter was fed its first solid food: a tender, young sacrificial grit."

Between the two of us — he with his Georgia genes and me with my North Carolina roots — the story grew faster than Pinocchio's nose. The meat from the grit was cooked, ground real fine, mixed with butter, salt and, for a real treat, "you pour a red eye or two over it."

We told them how some famous nutritionist — we'd forgotten the name, but they'd surely recognize it — had recently gotten a federal grant for extensive research on grits.

"You may have read about it in USA Today," I said.

They hadn't.

"The studies showed there to be some chemical in grits that stimulates dying cells in hair follicles. A group of prematurely bald sophomores at the University of Virginia volunteered to eat grits for breakfast every morning of winter term."

Both Boston and Philadelphia stopped chewing.

Which was a good thing because it's hard to concentrate when people next to you are putting uncooked orange fish into their mouths first thing in the morning.

"Do you watch Donahue?" I asked on a brilliant impulse.

They didn't.

"Then you probably missed the show where they had those sophomores on. They'd all grown a full head of hair. Chests, too. They even took off their shirts to prove it . . ."

Philadelphia finally fell: "Pass the grits."

Boston never bit.

But everybody knows they are full of beans.

BEING A LADY
IS NO SWEAT

Marilyn Schwartz says Princess Margaret may be true-blue royalty, but she'd never make it past rush at Ole Miss. Why? Because she was once seen puffing on a cigarette in public.

Schwartz, a feature writer for The Dallas Morning News, has the scoop on what it takes to be in the sisterhood of high society, Southern style.

According to her "Southern Belle Primer," people who serve dark meat in their chicken salad probably wouldn't be happy in the Junior League of Atlanta.

Unless you learn to curtsy so deep your head actually touches the floor, you can't be a Texas debutante.

And true Southern belles spray their fannies with glue to keep their bathing suits from riding up at country club poolsides.

I probably should hide Schwartz's book from my mother.

My mother didn't think the be-all and end-all of life was to be Queen of the Divine Rainbow, and she never once served finger bowls at her bridge parties. In fact, she doesn't even know how to play bridge. Not once was I ever sent to my room for not acting like "a Southern belle."

But she was very serious about my being a LADY.

My sisters and I couldn't just grow up.

We had to become LADIES.

A LADY is the archangel of orthodox Southern living, high priestess of p's and q's.

My mother, and her mother before her, worked day and night, leading their daughters along the paths of righteousness so we would grow up and become — not women, hush your mouth — but LADIES.

If we really wanted to do them proud, we would become REAL LADIES.

A woman is what you become if you aren't a Nice Little Girl. A woman is common. Tacky. Doesn't come from a Nice Family. Has Bad Habits. And, worst of all, a woman is uncouth.

Does that mean a LADY is couth?

Of courth.

A LADY never puts lipstick on in public or eats dessert with a salad fork. She doesn't wear anklets. Never says "yeah" or "uh-huh."

Doesn't sit with her feet apart or elbows on the table.

The spoon never hits bottom when a LADY stirs her tea.

She does not slurp.

Or talk with her mouth full. In fact, she makes absolutely no noise whatsoever when chewing or swallowing, and if she should ever, ever b-u-r-p, well, we just won't even talk about that.

She never wads up her napkin, and, before leaving the table, she always asks if she "may" — a LADY would not say "can" — be excused, even if she hasn't done anything wrong and even if she does not have to go to the bathroom.

Oops. I goofed. LADIES don't have to go to the bathroom.

They powder their noses.

When a LADY eats soup, she never dips her spoon toward herself. She never stuffs muffins in her purse, never eats off other people's plates.

A LADY has soiled clothes. A woman has dirty clothes.

Women sweat. A LADY perspires.

A LADY never wears ratty underwear because "you never know when you might be hit by a truck."

She doesn't chew gum, put her feet on the coffee table or wear T-shirts that say things. She never lets the sun set on a sink of dirty dishes, a dead flower arrangement, a tarnished sugar bowl, chipped nail polish or an unwritten thank-you note.

She doesn't answer the door in her bathrobe.

We are, of course, all human, but there are certain things a LADY never does in front of another living creature, pets included: Cut her fingernails, blow her nose, wear curlers in her hair, hiccup, cuss, snore or spit.

It's OK — thank goodness — for a LADY to be a little "broad" . . . but she better not ever talk like one.

SOUTHERN-FRIED SECRETS

I t's high time they made a movie about Southern food. Nowhere in the world is there such drama, such imagination, such enthusiasm about what to eat. Obviously, Southern cooking has nothing to do with where you eat it. It has to do with where it was thought up.

Fried green tomatoes are fried green tomatoes, whether eaten at a cafe in Alabama or a deli on East 58th, across from Bloomies.

For a long time grits was (were? ever seen a grit?) the staple of Southern foodism. Cigar-chewing, beer-gutted, slime-ball politicians and their ditwad blonds (in other words, all Southerners in every movie you have ever seen) were usually fixin' to eat a bowl of grits . . . a dead giveaway that they wouldn't have known a grit from a gumbo.

You don't eat a bowl of grits. You eat a mess of. Or a plate of. Or even a pot of.

Or else, you turned up your nose and said, "I don't like grits," which means there is something bad wrong with you.

Or your mama.

Until Hollywood discovered fried green tomatoes, it was mostly grits. Or mint juleps, sipped on verandas and piazzas one after another until the mosquitoes moved in for their supper.

We used to laugh at the tour guides in Charleston, S.C., who fed visitors lines like "Some of those itty bitty graves out yonder in the churchyard are little chil'run who died of hominy burns or brass polish inhalation."

They always got bigger tips when they talked like that.

But thanks to Fannie Flagg's book and Jessica Tandy's movie, folks are getting a broader perspective on Southern food.

I'm not sure it's such a good idea to let out too many secrets.

Think about, for example, what they'll do to peanuts once the world discovers that the best way to eat them is boiled.

Look what happened to popcorn.

Flavors.

Can you imagine cheese-boiled peanuts? Cinnamon-coated boiled peanuts?

And heaven help us if they discover what a pack of salted Lance peanuts can do to a Pepsi: tear it open with your teeth, pour it into a freezing cold bottle of Coke or Pepsi and . . . *mmmmmmhhhhhhm.*

Doesn't work with cans, and lordy only knows what it would taste like if they started doing it for you at the factory, calling it something like P-Kola or Cok-a-pea.

Aunt Jemima better hope they never make a movie called "Johnnycakes and Syrup on Sunday Nights at Home."

Waffles and pancakes are eaten only by people who don't know how to make cornbread.

Southern children have a knack for making up recipes. I personally knew the teenaged girls in Richmond who came up with the idea of putting potato chips in chocolate ice cream and stirring it up into a mush. Now folks are paying good money for such at Baskin-Robbins and TCBY like it was some great new discovery.

But as far as green tomatoes go, let's just let Hollywood know about the frying part.

Don't tell them about green tomato pickles.

Once they taste that, there's no turning back.

NATURE'S FLASHLIGHTS

Chicken Little wasn't all wrong. Sometimes the sky does fall. Especially on lazy Southern summer nights.

If you don't believe me, take a look out some night, just as the warm quicksilver of daylight slips off the horizon. You'll see it then: The night sky, all lit up with stars, falling into your own backyard.

Whole galaxies of twinkling lights, silently winking, blinking and nodding in a black sea.

Actually, they are lightning bugs. At least, that's what folks call them in North Carolina backyards.

Folks in some other places call them fireflies. Whatever you call them, a bug so magic it glows in the dark is surely one of the wonders of the world.

And of childhood.

Remember the first one you ever caught?

Getting up the nerve to close your fingers over the tiny, tickling thing and holding it — not too tight, not too loose — long enough to get it inside the mayonnaise jar before it died of suffocation or you smushed it to death?

The hardest part was how you had to lift off the lid just wide enough, then hold your hand at precisely the right angle so he'd kind of crawl in by himself.

Or herself, I suppose.

Remember the excitement of taking an ice pick and making holes in the top for him/her (how do you tell?) to breathe? In Georgia — so my husband says — no kid would be so cruel as not to throw in a little grass for food or comfort or for whatever lightning bugs do with grass. That would make them feel more at home in captivity.

In North Carolina, we just let them fend for themselves inside the jar.

Once a friend and I caught two huge Mason jars full and let them loose at the Manor Theater during the previews.

What a wonderful sight it was.

We'd gotten the idea from a cousin who lived in Atlanta and was always bragging about the Fox Theater where he went to the movies. The Fox Theater, we were never allowed to forget, had stars on the ceiling. Whenever he went to the movies, he could look up and it was like there was no roof. You could see practically all the way to heaven.

Well, we fixed it so that for one shining hour, the Manor Theater had stars everywhere. You didn't even have to look up.

And our stars twinkled.

It occurred to me the other night that, as a child, I never wondered how or why lightning bugs did what they did.

Only people without imagination, people who need to understand something in order to enjoy it, would ever ruin such marvelous, mysterious magic with something as dull — as irrelevant — as an explanation.

Now, look at me. I'm an old fuddy-duddy. I've actually gone to the encyclopedia, which, if you have any childhood left in you, is no place to enjoy lightning bugs.

(A chemical reaction in the dorsal prothorax, below the elytra in Lampyridae, especially the Photinus pyralis, produces, at peak, nocturnal bioluminescence at 1/50 candle power intensity — the interaction of luciferase, luciferin and adenosine triphosphate . . . Now you know what to tell the kids, should they ask.)

Personally, I think it's more fun to think of them as stars or fairy eyes or any of a thousand things more interesting than adenosine triphosphate.

Poets never get into the scientific stuff. How memorable would a song be if it went like this:

Glow, little Pyractomena ecostata, glimmer, glimmer,
Hey there! Don't get dimmer, dimmer . . .

Or, if Thomas Moore, in his ballad, had written:

They made her a grave, too cold and damp
For a soul so warm and true;
And she's gone to the Lake of the Dismal Swamp,
Where, all night long, by a photuris' bioluminescence,
She paddles her white canoe.

~ ~ ~ ~ ~

The $750,000 question is . . . where was Andrew Jackson's "hometown?"

North Carolina claims him, South Carolina claims him, and over in Nashville is a huge tourist set-up at The Hermitage — "Home of Andrew Jackson."

Then there is Florida, where he was governor; New Orleans, where he saved the day; and, of course, he once lived in Washington, D.C.

Jackson himself didn't seem to know for sure. He went on record claiming both Carolinas as his birthplace.

Does that mean he was born again?

A MAN OF STATURE

It might not impress an East Tennessean, but I was actually in Richmond, Va., for Robert E. Lee's birthday. If you are from Virginia, you know that means I was in the holy city for the birthday of a saint.

In fact, on the 19th of January, I visited the famous statue of Lee there on Monument Avenue, where about half a dozen good old boys all decked out in Confederate uniforms marched in serious formation underneath the general himself, posed astride his faithful horse, Traveler.

Virginians prefer that monument to other reincarnations of Lee because, in most portraits, Lee unfortunately has his hand on his hips in kind of a sissified pose that went over big with the English and French in days of yore but doesn't cut it with macho American military-types of today.

Believe me, that zillion-ton statue of Lee sitting tall on top of a gigantic Traveler is a sight to behold.

It wasn't Gen. Lee's birthday that took me to Richmond, but it was a birthday. One of Lee's staunchest admirers, namely my mother, turned 80 two days before Lee would've blown out 184 candles had he done what old soldiers are supposed to do and just faded away instead of actually dying.

As it is, any true Virginian would knock you upside the head if you ever so much as suggested that Gen. Robert E. Lee faded away into anything, even the musty pages of history.

It was a Saturday, and traffic was moving along smoothly on Monument Avenue. Mother and I drove past J.E.B. Stuart, A.P. Hill, Stonewall Jackson. We chatted about the things mothers and daughters chat about . . . but when we got to Lee on Traveler, we slowed the car down and observed a moment or two of respectful silence.

After all, it was not only Lee's birthday — it was Confederate Heroes Day, and in Virginia, that's like unto Christmas. Sort of.

I wouldn't be surprised if Lee's Birthday/Confederate Heroes Day wasn't written into church lectionaries in places like Arlington, Appomattox, Williamsburg and Richmond. (Did you know that there are more Episcopalians than people in Virginia? You might say Virginia is where Episcopalians are the densest. Of course, you'd never say that if you were Episcopalian, but Presbyterians are allowed to say it without having to do a whole lot of penance.)

Anyway, there we were looking up at Lee — on his birthday — with soldiers saluting crisply and walking stiff-leggedly around in squares on the steps beneath.

I remembered a story I heard about another intergenerational pair of Lee "worshipers."

The fellow in this story was lucky enough to have been born not only in Virginia, but also in its mecca — and he grew up on Monument Avenue. Over the years, he memorized all the old War Between the States stories (in Virginia it's never called the Civil War, and don't ask me why unless it's because Virginians are never uncivil, even to Yankees). He collected scads of those little cast-iron soldiers, turning his bedroom floor into Gettysburg, Bull Run or any place his little heart desired.

He went to Washington & Lee — where else? — and married a nice Richmond girl who sat a smooth canter and said "hoose" and "aboot," and before long they had a little cavalier of their own, a son they named Randolph or Cabell — I forget which.

Every Saturday, father and son visited the Lee statue on Monument Avenue, and the little boy heard history repeat itself. Then came the death blow.

The fellow was transferred to New Jersey.

The morning the moving van pulled out for the Far Country, his son asked to go visit Lee one last time. As they stood there in the rain, the little boy tugged at his father's coattail and said, "Dad, there's just one thing I've always wanted to know . . . who is that old man sitting *on* Lee?"

My mother sent me a napkin that says, "To be a Virginian either by birth, marriage, adoption, or even on one's mother's side is an introduction to any state of the Union, a passport to any foreign country and a benediction from the Almighty God."

A friend sent a postcard that reads, "If you live a good life, say your prayers and go to church . . . when you die, you get to go to Charleston."

Anybody ever read anything like that about Chicago?

VIII. ADVENTURES ELSEWHERE

The term "spirit of adventure" has become such a hackneyed, commercialized label it has lost its punch; but it is something we should take out and polish up, no matter how young — or old — we are. It keeps life from becoming vanilla.

My next time around, I want to be a photo-journalist for The National Geographic. Wonder what those people do when they are on vacation. Laundry? Go to the dentist? Grow mold in front of the TV?

Most of us don't have that problem. We hoard up our days off and have to choose among a thousand things we want to do. So much to do, so little time. Once you have been bitten by the travel bug, you're a goner. But you also discover that a love of adventure and travel is not a "bug" at all.

It's a blessing.

MOUNTAIN PEOPLE, BEACH PEOPLE

There are, basically, two kinds of people in this world: Beach people and mountain people. One takes the high road. One the low.

Of course, there's no right and wrong in all this. God made mountains and God made beaches and then gave us freedom to decide which way to point the car come vacation time.

Mountain people have patron saints like Heidi and L.L. Bean, Edmund Hillary . . . Alexander the Great.

Beach people have theirs: Jonathan Livingston, Captain Ahab, Jacques Cousteau . . . Popeye.

Some people can sit happily growing mold for hours, watching mountains do nothing but stare back. Put these same people on a terry cloth towel, watching waves do what they have done for millions of years

245

without changing their act one little bit, and they get itchy.

"The beach is muggy and hot, sandy, icky and buggy," say the mountain people.

"The mountains are wet, foggy, dark," says the beachcomber.

Which are you? When it comes to vacations, do you want your brain to melt or mildew? Think about it.

The mountains have poison ivy, copperheads, spotted fever, twangy music, hairpin curves and lousy TV reception.

Beaches have sand spurs, swimmer's ear, loud music, sharp shells and a sticky film of salt fogging up your glasses.

When you go to the mountains, you have to pack raincoats, fold and unfold road maps, pop Dramamine and watch for falling rocks.

When you go to the beach, everybody has to pack in one suitcase to make room in the car for sunscreens 1-100 and mega-strength bug spray, for rods and reels, electric fans, flyswatters, kites, rafts and every towel in the linen closet.

In the mountains, you sleep without sweating, listen to the rain sing on a tin roof, eat apples that sizzle when you bite into them, sending your taste buds into delicious agony. You take long walks and watch the sun shimmer on flecks of mica, turn ferns into diamonds and tickle the spine of mountain ridges straight out of "The Sound of Music."

You picnic beside streams with water so clear you have to put your feet in to make sure it's real. Afterward, nap between a four-poster of laurel underneath a canopy of rhododendron.

You stick to the sheets at the beach. Find sand in your toothpaste. You use up all the ugly words you know when the clouds move in and you have to lower every window in the house before it floats away.

The water tastes funny. You can never find all the kids and both your flip-flops at the same time. As soon as you get settled on your towel — after tap dancing across hot sand, hauling inner tubes and beach chairs — someone always has to go to the bathroom. Crayons melt on the dashboard and your face stays so oily your sunglasses ride off the end of your nose.

The mountains give you a sense of wonder and awe. They're full of stories and antique auctions, maple syrup and clogging.

The beach gives you hay fever and frizzy hair. It's full of

jellyfish and melted Chap Stick. There is never enough ice, too many ants and arcades.

Smelly bait in the freezer.

So.

What'll it be?

The beach. It's a close call — but the beach wins.

The beach is fishing pier mornings and Damascus Road sunsets and nighttime symphonies played beneath your window.

The beach is low-flying gulls brush-stroking a Mother-of-pearl sky, calling you down to watch the water stir from its sleep and roll out a new day. Tiny sandpipers that patrol on tiptoe along the edge. Sea oats fanning from the dunes.

At night, the sun is wound around in bright scarves until, like magic, it's gone.

The beach has low tide, when you can count the earth's ribs and walk through warm tidal pools, then sit in the inlet and have the world all to yourself.

Beach or mountains? It's almost a toss-up.

But not quite.

CHASING AFTER CHAUCER

Clipping along in my backward seat on the train from London to Canterbury, I am glad my mother warned me not to let anything hang out the window on moving cars, buses or rides at the fair.

Anybody who stuck her head out this half-cocked window for a breath of English country air would risk decapitation as we zoom through tunnels and under bridges.

The show changes every second:

A maze of row houses, with laundry dancing on the line, homegrown tomatoes and morning glorys marching right up to the back screen door.

A family of cows asleep in a pond.

A postcard scene of the Thames.

My train career is pretty much limited to all-nighters, coach class, from Richmond to Atlanta back and forth from college, sleeping on my laundry after scouting out the club car for guys.

There's something very basic about trains. The clackety-clack and mournful hoots tag your memories into a game of musical chairs. If you're not careful, you'll end up telling perfect strangers the story of your life.

Even imperfect ones.

You are so uninvolved in the responsibilities and mechanics of getting there, yet so unprotected from the jiggling and rocking, the smell of engine oil, the whoosh and whine of brakes and throttle.

There's a woman across the way, knitting, seldom looking down at the stitches. How does she do that? Doesn't she remind you of someone?

The expression on her face makes you curious and pensive as you watch her watch the patchwork fields whiz by. They, too, are stitched together in a haphazard way, puckered hollyhock meadows and tufts of tall grass sticking up like French knots.

A little girl across the way asks her mother where they are going. They drink out of the same paper cup and laugh at a secret I cannot hear.

We arrive right on "shed-ule," coming from Victoria Station to Canterbury in less time than it takes to get to an afternoon game on a football Saturday back home. Certainly faster than we could have made it had we rented a car and driven ourselves.

Besides, if we had driven, we'd all be dead on the side of the road from a head-on collision at the first roundabout. Nobody has yet explained to me why there are people in this world who drive on the left. I once hitchhiked my way through Ireland and Scotland, and it's a wonder I ever got where I was going because me and my thumb were always on the wrong side of the street.

By the time the train pulls into the station, I'm sorry I'll never know whether it'll be boys, girls or one of each who wear the white suits the woman is knitting. Her sister, she's told us, waited 10 years before having children, and now the doctor says it'll be twins. Due in six weeks. Caesarean, of course.

Along the way, we've picked up a group of knee-socked girls on a school outing, each one wrapped in the same plaid skirt and tied up in a white middy. Some have the zipper going up the front. Some tie the bow on the side. A few roll up their skirts at the waist, others pull it down on their hips till it scrapes their shoes.

Outward evidence of the yin and yang wars inside.

I wouldn't call riding a train a pilgrimage of Holy Grail dimensions, but it sure beats talking to yourself in the car. Or trying to unclog your ears and bite open the bag of peanuts on the airplane.

If Geoffrey Chaucer had tapped me on the shoulder and asked me for a tale as we rolled into Canterbury, I'd be hard-pressed to come up with one to match, say, the Miller's or the Cook's; and I never got close enough to the wife knitting the baby clothes to see if she had a gap in her front teeth; but I'll bet my train fare that behind the whispers and the giggles, the hopscotch of memories and the knit-one-purl-two that binds us all as humans headed for who knows where — there were some good stories we'll probably never hear.

~   ~   ~   ~   ~

Do you plan to take a vacation this summer? In 1954, when the Gallup Poll asked the question, 37 percent of Americans answered yes and 51 percent no. In 1991, 59 percent said yes and 36 percent no. When the stay-at-homes were asked why, 44 percent gave answers like cost / expense / money is tight.

Destinations of those vacations? Outside the United States, 12 percent. To another state, 66 percent. Within own state, 22 percent. Where outside the United States? Top three: Europe, Mexico, and Canada. The Soviet Union scored behind the Caribbean and the Bahamas, but ahead of Virgin Islands, Bermuda, Greece, Ireland, Israel and all of South America.

In domestic travel, the top five states were Florida, California, Colorado, South Carolina, and Virginia.

SCENT-AMENTAL JOURNEYS

Even in Birkenstocks, an old ragg sweater and hiker's hair — a mother is a mother is a mother. Despite my disguise, the seat-assigners at USAir knew a veteran of the trenches when they saw one, and I'm convinced that's why they put me, traveling alone on the long flight home from a rafting vacation on the Colorado River, between a 16-month-old and a 4-year-old, behind a 2-year-old, and across the aisle from an airsick father with an airsick toddler.

By the time I got home, I'd relived those nightmare trips in the car back when our kids were little. Taking them anywhere took courage, a sense of humor, a bag of bribes and a mental replay of our marriage vows.

"When are we gonna get there?"

"Make him stop picking on me."

"I'm hot."

"I'm cold."

"Mama, my mouth is watering. I feel sick."

And we wouldn't even be out of the driveway.

Like I said, motherly types seem to send off some kind of bleep. The kid in front knew I'd be a good sport when he reached over the seat, took a swat at my coffee cup and dumped it into my backpack.

The man across the aisle knew, somehow, that, yes, I would be glad to hold his child while he went to the bathroom and that, no, it wouldn't hurt my feelings when the kid looked at me like I was Jack the Ripper, screamed for me to let him loose, told the whole planeload of people that he did not like me and then threw up. On me.

The 16-month-old next to me knew that when she got tired of her grape juice and applesauce, she could just spit them in my lap. She even decided to put her chewing gum on my nose when it lost its flavor.

And when she lost her cookies, so to speak, she naturally looked my way.

It was a very rough flight.

But, then, traveling with kids is always rough. How many times can you sing "Little Rabbit Foo Foo" without going nuts? I remember well those endless drives to Georgia to spend Thanksgiving with my husband's family, way back when.

I'd beg him to let me drive. But, no.

"I don't mind," he'd say bravely.

When we finally drove in the driveway, my hair was pulled out by the roots, my lap sore from being jumped on, arms paralyzed from holding sleeping heads. Lollipops stuck to my shoes, game pieces and crumbs itched all down the front of my blouse, and nobody wanted to even touch the wet washrag we always traveled with.

Usually, whoever needed it had been sitting in my lap when they needed it.

My mother-in-law would take one look at us getting out of the car and get that poor-baby look on her face as she helped my husband to the door.

"Ohhhhhh. You look so tired, son. Come in and rest here on the sofa while Ina puts the children down, brings you some iced tea, fans your face, wipes your feet, pats your hand . . . you mean you drove all the way? I bet you are exhausted!"

I'm kidding, of course. It wasn't that bad. I really didn't have to fix the iced tea. Just bring it to him.

Once, when the children were something like 3, 5 and 6, even he lost it. They kept asking and kept asking "how much longer" and "are we almost there?"

After the eleven hundredth time, he turned around and pointed his finger while I grabbed the wheel: "DON'T ASK ME ONE MORE TIME HOW MANY MORE MILES OR IF WE ARE ALMOST THERE. JUST DON'T ASK."

Silence in the back seat. Absolute silence.

Then, a little voice:

"Dad? Just tell me this. How old will I be when we get there?"

I didn't actually grow old on my plane trip home from Arizona, but as I got my welcome-back hug, my husband wanted to know, "What's that smell?"

Why should he recognize it?

THEIR OLD
KENTUCKY HOME

In 1773, Daniel Boone led a party of
axmen who hacked their way along the
Wilderness Road through the
Cumberland Mountains. When he came
to the Gap — with its towering White
Rocks, its caves hidden in "hells" of matted
and relentless undergrowth — he wrote in
his journal: "The aspect of these cliffs is so
wild and horrid, that it is impossible to
behold them without terror."

The Cumberland Gap, where Kentucky,
Virginia and Tennessee meet in a tangle of
woods, a plunging river and jagged valley
basins, is steeped in history, much of it as
violent as the land is rugged. The Gap has
been a gateway through the mountains for
centuries. Referred to in history books as the
Warriors Path, it opened the way to Ohio at
the Scioto River, to the Carolinas by way of
the Catawba Trail, south to Chattanooga,

west to Middle Tennessee.

Fifth-graders from coast to coast have colored and labeled it on their history workbook maps and studied whole chapters devoted to its significance in the pioneering of America. A coveted hunting ground, a strategic battlefield, an area where cultures, nationalities and special interests clashed — the Cumberland Gap played out a tragic role in the lives of Indians and early white settlers.

Today, high on a plateau, hardly half a day's walk from the Gap, is a monument to the other side of that dark and bloody history. The mist lies like a blanket in the morning sun, apple trees offer their prized fruits to whoever wanders by, and the wind combs through grassy fields like fingers on a harp. The Hensley Settlement is a tribute to the human spirit, to peace and hard work, to self-sufficiency and devotion to, if not joy in, the simple life.

A hundred-fifty years before Sherman Hensley and his wife, Nicey Ann, moved to that remote mountain top in the Cumberlands, the 18th-century poet John Donne decided that "no man is an island, entire of itself . . . "

Donne might have had second thoughts had he visited the Hensley Settlement in its prime.

Sherman Hensley arrived in 1903, soon to be joined by other families: mostly Gibbonses and Hensleys. By 1925, the Hensley Settlement was at its peak, with more than 100 people living on what they produced and in what they built, remote and utterly withdrawn from even their closest neighbors, some eight miles down the rugged mountain.

There was no electricity. No automobile. No doctor. No store.

Today, in the neon glare of a rainy autumn afternoon, the voices of those that lived on this mountaintop "island" still speak, though the last inhabitant left in 1951.

There's the blacksmith shop. The houses chinked with mud. Bee stands. A foot-powered sewing machine. Dried flowers from long-ago Decoration Days.

Lige Gibbons said back then that the way to tell a man from a boy was by the amount he could carry from one side of the settlement to the other or up the primitive path from Virginia or down the Kentucky side along Brownies Creek. You can still see the sourwood sleds that were used to haul up supplies from far-off Caylor, Ewing and Cubbage.

Neal Robbins once carried up a hundred pounds of sugar.

Horse-drawn hay rakes, 70 acres of split-rail fences, the old gristmill, an empty schoolhouse, a wooden wagon and the smokehouse all speak in the silent afternoon of Willie Gibbons' ingenuity, Wallace Hensley's way with butchering and preserving, of children born and raised on the Hensley Settlement, most never leaving the mountain until they were teenagers.

The cemetery is a hymn to the thin edge they walked in those first few months and years of childhood without penicillin and pediatricians; to marriages that neither a hard life nor an early death could unhinge.

Some 37 people are buried there, the graves marked by fieldstones and understated tribute. Sherman Hensley has nine children buried on the mountain, Lige Gibbons, three.

In 1965, the Park Service began restoring the buildings that had deteriorated during the 1940s and early '50s as the old folks died off and the young folks left for college and jobs. Sherman Hensley — the first to arrive and the last to leave — lived there alone for two years before leaving the mountain in 1951. He said his old complaint about life on the mountain was that "the outhouse was too far away in the winter and too close in the summer!"

Today, in addition to running a shuttle bus to the settlement from its headquarters in Middlesboro, Ky., the Cumberland Gap National Historical Park maintains the buildings and fields. National Park Service Farmer Demonstrators use the Hensley Settlement as a teaching center, offering special events for tourists and school groups to see how tools were made, log houses were constructed, wild game was prepared and stored, quilts were sewn, and moonshine run on the side.

The restoration makes it easier to imagine and appreciate a style of life that is quickly passing from all living memory:

Reading by the light of pine splinters; sleeping on straw beds with rope bottoms; planting a field by moonlight. A time when the only medicine for tuberculosis and pneumonia and complicated birthings was prayer and what grew in the woods. When fires were put out bucket by bucket. When children had no time for boredom and invented their own games: Annie Over with a yarn ball or marbles with a shooter made from creek clay.

We bounce along the twisting road up from Middlesboro in the Park Service van, along Shillalah Creek, past kudzu creatures that nurse the mosquitos and tease the honeysuckle . . . watching leaves turn as dead as the tobacco drying in nearby barns down in the valley . . . feeling the first icy breath of winter, knowing that in a month or two, the woods would make nice Christmas cards, but hard, hard living . . . imagining what it would be like to carry a hundred pounds of sugar up to the top, or a dying child down for help . . .

One tourist from Georgia put into words what crosses everyone's mind on their way to the Hensley Settlement:

"People have to be playing with half a deck to want to live up here."

After the visit, one has to admit they may have lived off half a deck — but these people had all the aces.

A TRIP THROUGH TIME

Maybe seeing the ocean for the first time ranks up there with seeing the Grand Canyon for the first time. Maybe.

I don't remember a time when I hadn't seen the ocean, couldn't see it or hear it at the flick of a mental switch. But I can tell you the time, date and where the sun was in the sky when I first saw the Grand Canyon.

They say a picture is worth a thousand words, but no words or pictures prepared me for the jolt, the "Oh, my God" gasp for breath, as I walked out on the rim of the canyon that day.

My husband and I had flown to Albuquerque, then driven to the South Rim for a view from the top before we set out on a 230-mile white-water rafting trip on the Colorado River through the canyon. The next morning, we hiked nine and a half miles into the gorge on the Kaibab Trail, carrying everything on our back and a gallon of water to keep us alive in the 110-degree heat until we could lie, fully clothed and praising God, in water so cold it felt like fire.

We'd read everything we could find about the Anasazi, the Glen Canyon Dam, Vulcan's Throne, Havasu Falls and the rise of commercial river-running. We'd even looked at enough pictures in picture books to be able to recognize fishhook cactus and red-tailed hawks.

But nothing prepared us for what we saw and heard and felt.

How do biblical "literalists" explain things when they go to the Grand Canyon and read its creation calendar, left in no uncertain terms, in the layers of time set down like exhibits in a colossal, hands-on museum? Schist and gneisses, metamorphic rocks documented to be 2 billion years old, have been polished by rivers as old as time itself and shine like onyx in the inner gorge. Touching them is to relive the scene painted on the ceiling of the Sistine Chapel. It is a human and divine contact point.

We trace our fingers along fossilized reptile tracks from the Permian age, 230 million years ago. Footprints, literally, in the sands of time.

At every turn — on the river and in the visitors' center — is evidence of intelligent, spiritual, prehistoric life: the visible and invisible presence of desert cultures occupying the canyon hundreds and hundreds of years before any white man "discovered" it: Anasazi, Kayenta, Cohonino, Hualapai, Paiute, Hopi, Navajo.

The guides tell us the park service gets a number of letters a year from irate "six-day" Christians who take issue with our government for telling people the canyon is older than the numbers "allow" in the book of Genesis. But the canyon is just the place to go if you want to see the Creator. The wind plays the walls like pipes on an organ. At night, the stars light up like prayer candles, and sleeping on the warm sandy beach is like going back to the womb.

The rapids — some of the biggest runable white water in the world — speak of power and glory. Gliding along the quiet water, as it knifes its way through zoroaster granite and underneath stained-glass windows of redwall limestone and quartzite, you feel the fragile "forever and ever" of time as we can never know it.

As the sun moves across the floor of the canyon, the walls themselves seem to heave and sigh, changing personality and shape. In the early morning, they're stacked up like Legos. In the bright sun, they look like sleeping gods.

Toward evening, they change into dragons. At night, especially around a spooky-story campfire, you sit inside Dracula's castle.

But the canyon pulls at the spirit even more than the imagination, and after six days I have cracked the case. I know where I have been.

To God's workshop.

Probably the most potent artistic tool is the human eye. It can find pictures in the clouds, see oceans on the desert horizon and turn the night sky into a gallery of gods and goddesses.

The Grand Canyon is a blank canvas on which all sorts of stories have been "illustrated" in eye sculptures. Did you know that our own Dolly Parton has left her mark on the canyon walls? Our river guide told us the story and showed us the place.

Seems she got into this bungee jumping craze and took a leap off the rim above a turn in the river, just south of Saddle Horse Canyon. But, the cord broke and Parton landed upside the wall above us, leaving a sandstone imprint of her . . . er . . . person.

Two caves close together above a skinny waist.

It's not exactly a Rodin or da Vinci — but not bad for an on-the-spot eye sculpture.

THIS AIN'T NO BLARNEY

The summer of my sophomore year in college, a friend and I spent two weeks hitchhiking our way around Ireland.

We were, I am sure, the happiest wanderers that ever stuck out a thumb. We stayed in youth hostels, which back then cost about $1.25 a night and included a meal — usually fried bread and potatoes swimming in vinegar. But after hiking all day, it was delicious.

Three days before our flight out of Shannon, we ran completely and absolutely out of money. We spent our last nights counting sheep in a barn outside Limerick. If you are a logical person, you might want to know how come sheep were sleeping in a barn. I can't answer that. American sheep may sleep outside under the stars, but at least one farmer in Ireland bunks his in a barn.

He'd just finished tucking them in when we happened by and, looking over the situation, decided to borrow a little hay for the night. Nobody would be the wiser, and it wouldn't cost us a dime.

Sheep wake up real early. The only thing up any earlier is the shepherd — and there in the moonlight all we could see were two eyes and a pitchfork.

"You think 'tis a hotel, do you now?" came a voice that sounded like a tune played on a country fiddle.

The Irish are kindhearted people. Not only did he let us sleep in his barn the next two nights, he fed us enough oatmeal to pave an entire parking lot.

Time has swallowed up most of those names and faces from that vagabond summer, but never will it take with it the picture-postcard scenes I keep on file in my head for emergencies: Children with cheeks like polished apples sitting in the back of jaunting carts, hair bouncing and arms waving. The sun riding whitecaps on Dingle Bay. Our laundry spread out on the grass beside a creek in Ballybunion. Stone roads leading from nowhere to next-to-nowhere out on the Aran Islands.

But there's one night I wish I could forget.

It was early on, back when we had money to spend on fish and chips for supper, and afterwards cups and cups of hot tea with fresh cream. Lots of tea.

Which is what made the night so memorable.

We were at a youth hostel in County Mayo, on the western coast, overlooking Achill and Blacksod Bay. It was a very basic place. No electricity. No neighbors. Just a few boards some brave souls had nailed together there on the high cliffs, and it was only half-broke young people off on a dare who got up the nerve to spend the night so close to the edge. The hostel stood downwind from a fence of rocks that clung on for dear life in fear of dropping to the roaring sea below.

There's no way to describe what it looked like. Any attempt seems a sacrilege.

I think of it as a place where God decided to do something different. Taking pinking shears out of the drawer, he reached over into the pile of creation cloth, pulled out every shade of green velvet he could find and cut out little squares. He took burlap, rumpled it up to look like rocks worn smooth by winds from the four corners of time. He unrolled a bolt of blue taffeta sky, then sprinkled the whole thing with sequins to catch the sun. Or the moon. Or even the imagination.

If all this seems like too much overdone poetry and exaggeration — then I might be getting close.

Anyway, we were spending the night in this magic place, where you could see pieces of creation lying all around.

We sat up way into the night, talking and drinking hot tea. I know the Irish have a reputation for drinking more than tea, but we were early risers with lots of walking ahead of us. Tea bags weigh nothing in a backpack, so it was the drink of preference for many reasons.

During the night I had to do what people who drink lots of tea have to do in the middle of the night. The outhouse was a separate building, down a path toward the edge of the cliff. I took my flashlight, buckled up my courage and off I went. I won't go into great detail here, but the outhouse consisted of a deep ditch and a board, to put it bluntly. There was a latch on both the outside and the inside because the wind came through that place like a train making up time, so the door had to be secured from the outside when leaving.

It was not my lucky night.

Suddenly, the wind hit the side of that outhouse like nothing you've ever heard. It scared me so bad I dropped my flashlight into the — uh — ditch. Then, it shook the door so hard, the outside latch fell across, locking me inside in the dark . . .

It was a long night. Evidently no one drank as much tea as I did.

I recited Shakespeare. I sang all the verses of every camp song and hymn I knew, and I swore up and down that if the Good Lord would get me out of that fix, I would be a saint on this earth forever and ever.

Even after all these years, I refuse to go into outhouses. You couldn't get me back in one for all the tea in China.

Or Ireland.

HIKING THE CHIMNEY TOPS

Climbing the Chimneys is not for chickens. Some would say it's not for humans, either, but if you can talk yourself into it, it will be a sales job you won't regret.

Every clump of mountains has some peak or some trail that is known for its blisters, backbreaking challenge and breathtaking view. In North Carolina, it's Mount Mitchell. In Virginia, Mount Rogers. In Nepal, Mount Everest.

For us in the Smokies, it's the Chimneys.

Climbing the Chimneys is a rite of passage for people around here. It's also the Day of Reckoning, the Incredible Journey and a time when your whole life is likely to pass before your eyes. Going up is a test of stamina, of the treads on hiking boots and of the pull of gravity. Coming down is a challenge to your rear end, your calf muscles and your panic button.

For at least one middle-aged, God-fearing mama it was as close to meeting her Maker as she plans to get until she sails off into the sunset on the last adventure of all. But for anyone over the age of accountability and younger than the last hurrah, it is wonderfully do-able.

When you get up the mountain to the base of the actual Chimneys, it seems unthinkable to go any farther, but, after a short rest and a canteen of water, there comes a second wind. Going out on a limb is one thing. Going out on a rock thousands of feet above sea level is something else.

Never mind how kids in their teens and 20s do it while having intelligible conversations with each other. For some goatlike people, it's a piece of cake. For others of us, it's huffing and puffing, swearing and praying and — at last, at the top — shouting so loud there's an echo across three valleys.

If your idea of fun is not to scale up polished slate while humming "Nearer, My God to Thee" — the view from the base is almost just as beautiful as from the top and certainly worth the climb.

All the books rate the hike to the Chimneys as "strenuous." Believe them.

It's a vertical rise of 1,350 feet in two miles to the Chimneys. The rock-climb to the top is straight up. Up up, as in "Oh, God, will we ever get there?" That is not meant as an oath. If you are like me, by the final leg-up and the last fingers-searching-for-a-hand-hold on the rock face, you'll be on a first-name basis with the Almighty.

The hike (that's what they call it, but it's more like a haul) to the base of the polished slate Chimneys themselves is sweetened with mountain laurel doing its thing, oxalis dancing underfoot and rhododendron flirting at every turn.

The well-used trail several times crosses a creek that wrote the book on what mountain streams are supposed to look like. The mossy, minty, mixed-up-green smell of the mountains works like incense on the soul and gives you a jump-start just when you think you're gonna die.

As you approach the Chimneys' parking lot — look up (unless

you are driving the car) and you'll get a preview of what you're getting yourself into . . . or, more exactly, up on. The Chimneys are the high, steep, span of rock overlooking the Sugarlands. You can't miss them. Unless they've got their face stuck in a cloud. Carry a day pack with snacks, a water bottle, a small camera and — if you're not accustomed to making up your own — the Book of Common Prayer.

Just kidding.

It's really not that bad. But climbing the Chimneys is one of those adventures that gets taller and taller every time you tell it. Part of the fun is bragging about how brave and strong you are to have done it.

If it rains, stay home.

Before you go, be sure and cut your toenails. Coming down is so steep, your feet slide forward so far they almost poke out of your shoes. And don't forget to thank your lucky stars for being healthy enough and smart enough for just doing it.

VROOOOOMMM VROOOOOOOOMMMM

Motorcycle madness is not congenital. As far as I know, I am the only person in my family who has it.

"Anybody who rides half a block on one of those things is ca-raz-zee" is the nicest thing my family has to say about the whole idea.

So, I was not blood kin to any of the 8,000-10,000 two-wheeling madmen (madpersons?) saddling up their Honda Gold Wings and Yamaha TDM850s at the annual Rider Rally outside the Grand Hotel in Pigeon Forge. The whole place looked like a wasp nest.

My vote for best bumper sticker was: "Remember when sex was safe and motorcycles were dangerous?"

Nothing will jump-start your heart quite like a hairpin curve — you know, the kind

where the taillights you see in front of you are your own! — with
the wind in your face and the world spread out like a wraparound
movie screen.

Just sit yourself down on a sheep-skinned custom seat . . . rest
your back against the plush leather upholstery . . . turn on the
stereo tape player . . . rev up them hush-hush Honda horses . . .
and put it on cruise control. It's like sitting in a vibrating La-Z-Boy
and watching a National Geographic special all at the same time.

Nobody should pass from this world without hearing "Ode to
Joy" sung by the Mormon Tabernacle Choir as you are riding the
Blue Ridge Parkway. Or "Waltz of the Flowers" through the
Smokies and over to Maggie Valley. I know Tchaikovsky never
rode a motorcycle, but bluets and daisy fleabane actually do a fast
waltz as you pass by.

On a motorcycle you see things you'd miss in a car: the
expression on a scarecrow's face, red eyes growling at you inside a
tunnel, what a multi-personality the color green has. The
underside of the Dillard Paper Co.'s 18-wheeler as you ride along
side-by-side on the interstate, the belching of an oil rig close on
your heels, and you're caught in a small tornado blowing off the
moving van in front of you . . . But we won't go into that, and don't
tell my family.

As often as I have crawled through Gatlinburg in a car,
cussing the jaywalkers and twiddling the steering wheel in
weekend traffic, I never noticed that telephone wires look — on a
pretty day — like struts and strings on a blue ukulele. All zipped
up in a car, you can only watch the fellow cutting the grass. You
can't smell it. If you didn't have to stop and stretch so often, you
might not pull off at the overlooks to make sure the mountains
really haven't turned into volcanos. It's just early morning fog.

The view from a motorcycle isn't put in a frame. You're part of
the painting. The needle-sharp steeples of country churches don't
get cropped off. You see the pattern pieces for shadows that cut
across valleys. You hear waterfalls. Watch reruns in two rearview
mirrors at once. Feel the road come untied beneath you like a
crinkly ribbon. A telephoto lens slips over your eyes, turning pink
rhododendron into scoops of raspberry sherbet, garnished with
mint.

Wide-angled views along the ridges near Clingmans Dome

give you a bird's-eye view of things. A hummingbird.

You feel like a hawk with a motor.

On the stairway to heaven at Waterrock Knob, talking to God is a local call.

I've never particularly cared for "Bolero" — Maurice Ravel's way of saying "Ole!" It sounded like a new piece to me as we kept time to it, leaning first one way, then another, on our way home along Newfound Gap Road. I played like the green leaves overhead were lace petticoats on a Spanish dancer's skirt. Fire pinks were buttons on a matador's cape.

Motorcycles, I guess, really do drive you crazy.

But what a way to go.

STEPPING INTO SCRIPTURE

We're sitting on bits and pieces of fallen columns and tumbled ruins in the marketplace where once upon a time the Apostle Paul stood.

Ancient Corinth is a ghost town now. The only voices you hear are tourists with maps and brochures, trying to get it all straight.

Where is Apollo's temple?

Which missionary journey was Paul on?

Why do so many religions and cultures come together here?

Paul traveled, we are told, to this wealthy, Roman town in the Peloponnese sometime during 51 A.D. Corinth then was the capital of the Roman province of Greece called Achaia. It was a strategic maneuver in the spread of the Gospel. But historians feel there was yet another reason Paul was determined to make the long journey: It was also the center of the Jewish community in this part of ancient Greece.

Our group of 28 "pilgrims" has chosen this spot to have a short reading and to celebrate Holy Communion. There are not many other tourists around, most preferring the beaches at New Corinth and the health spa in nearby Loutraki. Even for history buffs, the ruins in Ancient Corinth are more remote and less spectacular than up the road at Mycenae, where Agamemnon's sky-top citadel with its Cyclopean walls whisper stories stretching back 5,000 years. But for Christians, Ancient Corinth is a special place.

We take a linen hand towel from our hotel and spread it on a rock. The wine is poured into a juice glass borrowed from the breakfast table. The two soft rolls come from the cafe at the last rest stop. After reading the familiar words, we silently file by to dip the bread into the wine, taking it back to our places for silent prayer.

We're mostly Presbyterians. A few Episcopalians, a Roman Catholic and a Greek Orthodox keep us "honest." Many come from Baptist, Methodist or some other denominational background, so we have a variety of places and faces to associate with Paul's famous letter to the church here at Corinth some two thousand years ago: *Though I speak like an angel, though I understand every mystery, though I give my body to be burned . . . and have not love . . . I am nothing.*

Someone takes a handful of clover and wild grasses and fashions a cross, laying it on the cloth as she comes forward for communion. Nobody says much. At least, not out loud.

Later we talk about some of our thoughts:

How places can give shape and form to words.

How sharing something important can make us feel part of each other's lives, part of history, even part of some great plan we do not know but feel we can trust.

How never again will we read or hear the familiar words of I Corinthians 13 without coming back to this place, this moment.

I wonder what Paul would have thought, were he here among us. Maybe he is.

Does he approve?

We women do not have our heads covered. Not one of the men

has a beard. We have not pooled all our money. We do not share a common bank account. A number of women — if not all — speak out in churches back home as Sunday school teachers, elders, deacons, vestry officers. Paul didn't have much use for women and felt they should walk in the shadows and keep quiet. Especially in church.

He also pointed out that we see through a glass darkly in this world. Some things do change, even in religion.

"Words cease," wrote Paul to those who used to live in this place. "Knowledge vanishes."

But here in Ancient Corinth, at this moment, we share a faith and a hope that abides, that passes the tests of time. We feel among us a love that is stronger than these fallen stones.

THOMAS EDISON'S LAST BREATH

L ong before I'd ever been to Tennessee, I read about it on the sides of barns up and down highways from Richmond to Atlanta: "See Rock City."

By the time I actually saw Rock City, I was somewhat of a connoisseur of tourist traps.

There's nothing wrong with tourist traps. In fact, reptile farms, mystery hills, lost caverns and mummy museums are a whole way of life being paved over by interstates that take us places so fast we don't know where we've been.

Even the cows we used to play "poker" with on long trips are over the hill and out of sight. We travel anonymous, no-nonsense racetracks, edged by trees and chain-link fences. The places we make our pit stops have everything in common, a *deja vu* lineup of

BPs, Exxons and Quik Stops.

Gone are the giant spider signs, luring travelers into Tarantula Land . . . the lineup of cypress knees tempting us to see for ourselves the face of George Washington in a 300-year-old cross-section from the Okefenokee . . . the world's-largest-whatever (shrimp, prairie chicken, Indian mound) that no one with an ounce of curiosity or a carload of kids can drive by. We cruise-control around towns on beltways designed to get us from place to place without actually going through anything on the way. It's safer. It's more convenient. It's faster.

It's boring.

What about those "last chances" to see the "only fur-bearing trout in the world" (Wall, S.D.) . . . the house made of Fresca bottle tops (Arcola, Ill.) . . . God's Phone Booth (Crestview, Ky.) . . . the world's largest Duncan Phyfe Chair (Thomasville, N.C.).

Without such good old tourist traps to give us some place to go while we are going some place, well, if I were a kid today, I'd probably pester my parents to death asking and asking and asking: "Are we there yet?"

I cannot imagine going to Myrtle Beach without stopping at South of the Border, the great-granddaddy of all junky tourist attractions, there just over the line between my home state of North Carolina and its southern sister. You haven't seen roadside America at its finest until you've pulled up beside the neon sombrero and turned the kids loose to make up their minds whether to hit you up for a back scratcher, the salt and pepper shaker cacti or the velvet paintings of Bambi.

It was only a matter of time before somebody came up with an encyclopedia of such tourist traps, and I'm proud to say South of the Border is the lead article and got its picture on the front cover.

Tennessee scores well, too. Besides Rock City in Chattanooga, "Roadside America" lists 18 other Tennessee attractions as being among the wonders of the tourist world. Most of them are in — surprise! — Gatlinburg.

My favorite Tennessee tourist treasure along these lines is Graceland. It brings a lump to your throat to walk past the low-tide-green shag carpet in the King's Jungle Room, its leopard lampshades and zebra sofas just as he left them. The guide will tell you in a holy whisper that this is where the world-weary Elvis recorded his last two albums.

The Graceland gift shops are mind-boggling.

As "Roadside America" puts it, no souvenir better captures an Elvis devotee's tasteful reverence than the pastel blue, fuzzy bedroom slippers with plastic figureheads in true-to-life flesh tone.

With earmuffs to match.

When we were there, my husband made the awful mistake of asking in a stage whisper, "What was his daughter's name? I forgot."

But you have to remember: This is a guy who just said no when the kids asked if he'd buy them a windup monkey in the Natural Bridge gift shop, a year's supply of magic rocks at Waltzing Waters or the whoopee cushion at Weeki Wachee.

I'll have to hide "Roadside America" from our children, because — big as they are — they'll want to see Spongeorama (Florida), the Chalk Pyramids (Kansas), Jesus in a Bathtub (South Dakota), and the Giant Twine Ball (Minnesota).

Me? I can't wait to go to Michigan to see Thomas Edison's last breath. It's there, in a test tube at a museum outside Dearborn.

IX. . . . FROM THE BACK OF THE CLOSET

These are the misfits. The leftovers. They don't belong in any of the other chapters. It was even hard to think of a name to call the chapter they would be lumped together in. Somehow "Miscellaneous" didn't have much of a ring to it. We thought about "From the Back of the Fridge," which I thought was great until Susan Alexander pointed out that, with a name like that, it sounded like something green and furry that might make you sick. Closets, she said, hide as many treasures as they do trashables.

So we decided on "closet" instead of "fridge," although there is NO TELLING what you would find in the back of my closet. No one has looked in there for years.

WHAT'S IN A NAME?

What has (at least) two Mountains, twelve Hills, a heap of Valleys, four Groves and a handful of -ports?

The Tennessee Council of Teachers of English has come out with a nifty little booklet that explains, in alphabetical order, the names of places in Tennessee.

Ever heard of Yum Yum? Rattle and Snap? Stupidville? U Bet?

It's a drive-yourself-crazy book of blank verse, and it inspired me to tackle the post office's listings of place names in Tennessee. Sticking my head in those two books was like drowning in a delicious bowl of alphabet-city soup.

There's one Lowland, three Highlands, a Midway and more than four Corners.

I can't even count the "views" — just Lookout and Seymour.

If you think there is something fishy here, there is: Bass Landing, just for starters.

Then there's Soddy-Daisy, Tulip Grove, Cloverdale.

We've got Old Hometown, Fowlkes. Sweetwater and Stinking Creek. Counce and Crump. Eads and Eaton. Burns, Cookeville and Bakewell.

Speaking of food, Yuma. There's Jellico, Hoecake, Bean Station, Fruitvale, Riceville, Olivehill, Strawberry Plains and Sugar Tree. Ridgely, Beechnut, Chewing and Gum Station.

Hotland and Coalfield. Oldfort and Newport. Guys and Halls. Royal, Loyal and Doyle. Dickel and Tracy.

There's Cedar Hill, Hickory Withe, Peeled Chestnut, Piney Flats, Cypress Inn and Laurel Bloomery. Oaks have a -dale, a -hill, a -field, a -land and a Ridge.

There's Smart and Nutbush.

You may be more of a world traveler than you think. Look at all the places you can go without crossing the state line: Athens, Belfast, Brazil, Cairo, Denmark, Egypt, Lebanon, Memphis, Milan, Moscow, Normandy, Paris, Persia or Quebeck (we spell it our way).

And you can stay right here in Tennessee and still go to Charleston, Chapel Hill, Raleigh, Charlotte, Savannah, Macon, Philadelphia, Dayton, Cleveland, Santa Fe, Hollywood, Camelot.

And there are Lutts, Morley.

We've got just about every town in the rainbow: Brownsville, Graysville, Yellow Mountain, Auburntown, White House, Blue Bank, Silver Top, Red Boiling Springs. Green wins with Green Hills, Greenback, Greenbrier, Greeneville, Greenfield, Green Row and Moss.

There's Trust and Liberty. Trade and Prospect.

There's Parsons Branch, Church Hill, Cross Plains, Gilt Edge and Graceland. A trio of Saints: Andrew, Elmo and Joseph.

And a town called Baptist.

We've got Bulls Gap, Crab Orchard, Buffalo Valley, Deer Lodge, Panther Creek, Pigeon Forge, Turkey Creek, two Frog Hops and a Frog Town, an Owl City, an Owl Hoot and a Sheep Ridge.

There's Hollow Rock, Iron City, Limestone, Glass, Flintville, Cokecreek, Coalmont and Ozone.

Defence and Depot. Norris, Morris and Horace. Ten Mile, Two Forks, Five Points and Lone Mountain.

Sevierville and Wilder.

East and Eagan. Adams and Eva. Erin and Erwin, Marian and Marion. Maryville and Burrville (pronounced the same, but two different cities).

There are a jillion "sons," but no "daughters." Be that as it may, there are more towns with women's names than men's.

Arnold, Arthur, Chuckey, Giles, Henry, Lamar and Stewart as opposed to Celina, Lucy, Orlinda, Lavinia, Norene, Daisey, Sharon, Shirley, Viola, Bessie, Hortense, Isabella, Madie and Rhea.

As a body, we've got Finger, Skull Bone, Brainerd, Hartsville, Manchester, Reelfoot, Sweet Lips, Puryear, Gallaway and Farragut.

Harriman and his Harrison.

There's Holly Grove, Christmastown, St. Bethlehem, Holiday City, Garland and Gift.

Most names make sense when you hear their story.

There's only one Only.

One mountain community couldn't agree on what to tell the Post Office when asked to choose "a proper address."

"Forget the durn Post Office," shouted one take-charge sort of guy after days of heated debate. "This here's a nameless place if I ever did see one, so let it be."

And so it was. Is.

Nameless.

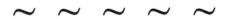

What is the only four-letter word in English that, when printed in capitals, reads the same upside down as it does right side up? You're getting warm . . . warmer . . . really hot . . . at NOON.

THE LAST BROADCAST

On Oct. 30, 1938, word came to the little town of Henderson, N.C., that everybody's worst nightmare was actually happening.

The Martians had not only landed, they were invading with such "express-train speed" that the National Guard, the Army Air Corps and New York City itself had been wiped out in half an hour.

People in Henderson had two choices on Sunday nights. If they weren't at church, they were around the radio, listening to either CBS's "Studio One" or Edgar Bergen and Charlie McCarthy on the "Chase and Sanborn Hour."

Services at Henderson's First Presbyterian Church had just let out. My father was on his way home, my mother busy putting two kids to bed, so the first they heard about the annihilation of New Jersey was when the phone started ringing.

"Shouldn't we hold a special prayer service?" someone called to ask.

My father was the minister of the First (and only) Presbyterian Church in Henderson, the person lots of people would want to talk to during the end of the world, so he counseled best he could while my mother turned on the radio.

The news had broken about 8:10 or so, during a commercial on the Edgar Bergen show. People have always played with the dials during commercials, so when the Chase and Sanborn people came on, little needles all over America roamed up and down the airways — until they came to "Studio One" and the voice of Carl Phillips, an actor cast as a news announcer in Orson Welles' radio dramatization of H.G. Wells' "War of the Worlds."

Phillips was doing a great imitation of Herb Morrison's voice the time Morrison eyewitnessed the explosion of the Hindenburg in what is now classic newscaster hysteria.

When my father turned on the radio that memorable Sunday night, Phillips was describing the Martians as they waded across the Hudson River:

"This is the end now . . . thousands of (people) dropping like rats . . . Now the smoke's crossing Sixth Avenue . . . Fifth . . . 100 yards away . . . 50 feet . . . "

Then the mike went dead.

Orson Welles was the furthest thing from Chicken Little as the eye can behold, but that night he convinced America that not only was the sky falling, but we'd been overtaken by flame-throwing Martians "tall as skyscrapers" whose black eyes gleamed "like a serpent" and whose "V-shaped" mouths had "saliva dripping from rimless lips that seem to quiver and pulsate."

Kinda gives you the creeps just reading stuff like that. Imagine hearing it as live-action news from, say, a spooked-up Peter Jennings.

Meanwhile, in the real world, phone lines were jammed, churches and bars were offering prayers and drinks on the house, stores were being looted, traffic jammed. Folks even contemplated suicide, because as one Pittsburgh woman found crouched in the bathroom clutching a bottle of poison put it: "I'd rather die this way."

A Nazi party newspaper blamed the Jews.

An Italian newspaper said "a third-grade democracy" had fallen into confusion.

The New York World-Telegram said if so many people could be misled unintentionally, no telling what could happen if "designing politicians" put their minds to it.

CBS called the show "regrettable." Orson Welles apologized publicly.

And whenever my parents told the story, it was always followed by a sermon on logic and crowd control — and, following that, a whole slew of stories about how wonderful life in Henderson had been, before television and bought fried chicken at church pot-luck dinners . . . and three more children.

~ ~ ~ ~ ~

When Thailand Television added "Laverne and Shirley" reruns to their regular schedule of programs, network officials knew that the idea of single women living away from home would be a cultural atrocity. People would never buy it. To avoid such an unthinkable premise, they begin each show with a statement that Laverne and Shirley have escaped from an insane asylum.

DOOR NO. 1 OR DOOR NO. 2?

Have you ever stood in the hallway outside a rest room in some restaurant and tried to decide which door to pick?

It used to be so simple: His. Hers. Ladies. Gentlemen. Men. Women.

Then things started getting complicated.

The trendy thing was to spruce up the names of everything.

Raw fish became sushi. Clabber became yogurt. Bean seeds and scum were passed off as sprouts and tofu.

And with nouveau cuisine came nouveau latrine.

First it was Lads and Lassies, Guys and Dolls, Jack and Jill.

Easy enough.

But then things went out of control.

Some restaurants figured that since a picture is worth a thousand words, they would rip off the words on the door and stick up pictures.

You had to choose between a face with hair growing over the lips or over the forehead.

Or maybe one with long, curly hair, one with a crew cut. Which led a lot of little kids astray if Dad's hair was longer than Mom's.

So they tried pictures of people wearing pants or skirts, hats or bonnets — which was also very misleading because some women seldom wear dresses, men no longer wear hats and nobody would be seen dead in a bonnet.

So they went back to words.

But not anything so dull and reasonable as Men and Women.

The words they use now — you need a dictionary to get it right.

A recent Dear Abby column took on Texas and its zeal to have everyone thinking Western, even when they go to the rest room. That can be a problem for city slickers who don't know right off-hand the difference between Heifers and Bulls, not to mention children whose stuffed animals aren't always anatomically correct.

One restaurant even tried Cows and Bulls, but a lot of women — even Texas women — felt insulted.

Family steak houses made going to the rest room risky business. Suddenly there was a steak house on every corner, every interstate exit. The menu was basically the same: silver-wrapped, 6-pound potatoes piled high with sour cream and plastic bacon; squares of red Jello with a Matterhorn of spray cream; beef in all its disguises, brought miraculously to the right table by cowgirls in brown and yellow checks.

The only difference in one steak house and another is the name on the door of the rest room: Senors and Senoritas. Fellers and Gals. Bucks and Does. Braves and Squaws.

Next, French restaurants went a la mode. They painted over the Ladies and Gentlemen with things like Mssrs and Ms or Demoiselle and Garcon.

All of which can get people who took Latin in trouble. Or anyone else who doesn't know a Le from a La — especially when in a hurry.

Indian restaurants can really mess you up since most of us don't know whether we're a Bibi or a Baboo.

Seafood places have Buoys and Gulls. Outboard and Inboard. He Crab and She Crab.

There's no telling what's ahead in the nouveau latrine business.

Italian restaurants could go Lasagnum, Lasagna. Masta or Pasta. The Colonel might tag his Roosters and Biddies.

Burger King could go Ferdinand and Daisy.

Po' Folks can keep the redneck-chic theme with Billy Goats and Nannies or Studs and Broads or Porky and Miss Piggy.

For the Chinese, there's always that old dilemma between yin and yang. Crystal Cathedrals and Heritage Villages could make it Samson and Delilah on the bottom floor, Angels and Archangels on the top.

MUCH ADO
ABOUT WILLIAM

Methinks it odd — anon, verily and hark — that Shakespeare was buried on his birthday.

For truth.

A day that appeareth on English exams for betrodden freshmen and celebrating seniors alike, for 'twas on April 23, 1564, that heaven sent down a poet and scholar bedeck'd with tongue so silver and pen so golden that all of history doth bend double before his books.

Upon Avon's Stratford it was that half a dozen pounds of flesh was deliv'd by the birthing bird to a glove maker and a farmer's daughter.

They called their son William.

Thirty-six plays and 164 sonnets later, at age 52, William was buried in Stratford parish church on April 23.

A poet by any other name would have

been easier to spell. He shaketh the spear of every sharp-spelling, cross-eyed ninth-grader who — like my own forefathers — forgetteth to add the "e."

Kings and clowns, meaner folk and students alike have furrowed their brow to cull the crop of keen insight deep within his verse.

I myself have cursed the darkness while burning the bewitching-hour oil, trying to pierce the cocoon to find the larva of truth, to spot the nits and gnats of iambic ironies that swarm within his plays like no-see-ums on a midsummer night.

As for English majors of any tongue, many hath watched night's candles burn out before jocund day stood tiptoe on a misty 8:30 — egad! — lit. class.

Children of an idle brain swear he wrote much ado about nothing. But when, perchance, a mind catches that life-giving pollen carried by winds of time and luck inside a good teacher's class, it stands in awe at the magic wand he waves over the alphabet.

He wrote about two Richards, two gentlemen, four Henrys, an emperor, a prince, a merchant, a god, a boudoir of merry wives, a campfire of witches and a center ring of half-wits that outwit us all.

His plays are performed all over the globe, actors and actresses strutting across the stage in a winter's tale, a summer's dream or some other story that passes with flying colors the test of time and season.

He taught us that parting is such sweet sorrow, that love is blind, that all the world's a stage and that the best way to spill the beans is to protest too much.

He warned us not to trust a man who has no music in his soul, not a borrower or a lender be, never to tempt a desperate man and bade us not to swear, but if we must, swear by ourselves and not by God.

He said only a fool would sell eternity for a toy.

He talked about the pink of courtesy, the purple of bleeding war and saint-seducing gold.

He asked a lot of questions:

Who is Sylvia? Et tu, Brute? Romeo, Romeo! Wherefore art thou?

Some we're still trying to answer, like whether we should suffer the slings and arrows of outrageous fortune in silence or rise up against a sea of troubles.

He taught us that youth's the stuff that will not endure and that good deeds are a candle in a naughty world. He said that, in life, one had to sink or swim and that death was like sleeping.

Sometimes he made us laugh at the wrong things, but it wasn't a comedy of errors. He brought back ghosts to coach the living.

"Nothing," he wrote "can we call our own but death and that barren earth which serves as paste to cover our bones."

His own epitaph reads:

Good friend for Jesus' sake forbear

To dig the dust enclosed here;

Blest be the man that spares these stones,

And curst be he that moves my bones.

Personally, I think he could have come up with something with a little more zip than that as his swan song.

Something catchy like "All's well that ends well." Or "Out! Out! Brief Candle!" Or "Goodnight, Sweet Prince. May troops of angels speed thee to thy rest."

Or maybe just a rousing "Forsooth."

For truth.

REMEMBERING ELEPHANTS

Until the circus came to town, I thought a pachyderm was something you chewed to get a good bubble.

But no.

A pachyderm is something that leads parades, will never have a perfume named after it, looks like it was made of leftover parts.

. . . and is very, very large.

The press kit Ringling Brothers and Barnum & Bailey sent told everything about elephants you'd ever want to know — except why anyone whose name is not Alex Gautier or Gunther Gabel-Williams would actually volunteer to ride one.

For me, the answer is simple: I'll do anything that makes me look small.

Sitting atop Siam, the 12,000-pound lead elephant, I look like a rag doll, flopping side

to side as Siam galuumps-galuumps-galuumps from the train
station, through the middle of downtown, across the interstate and
into the Civic Coliseum.

Siam has a face only a mother could love, but we all know
beauty is skin deep.

And Siam's beauty is well encased.

The first thing I notice about Siam close up is, in fact, her
skin. If she were human, she'd be an electrologist's nightmare.
Jergens lotion could make a killing on a pack of skin-conscious
elephants. I had on thick jeans and I still itch! It's like sitting on a
mountain of Fuller brushes. A moving mountain.

How do you get on and off an elephant? I was a little worried
about that at first. I thought maybe they'd have to get a cherry
picker to hoist me up and on. But Siam was very obliging. She just
knelt down, batted her tiny eyes underneath those wire lashes,
and said, "Giddyup."

Which I did, and praise be, landed up there in the right place.
One moment I was upside down in the air, the next I was coming
in for a landing on a great gray cactus.

How do you get down from an elephant?

You don't get down from an elephant, dummy.

You get down from a goose.

$\sim$ $\sim$ $\sim$ $\sim$ $\sim$

*Wanna be a real blue blood? Then you'll
have to be a lobster. Their blood is actually
blue.*

*And while we're seaing about things, a
shrimp's heart is in its head.*

WHY DINOSAUR EGGS ARE EXTINCT

I nearly had a heart attack the other day in the grocery store when I saw the price of watermelon. They wanted $5! Not that a good, cold watermelon isn't priceless, worth every cent you pay and all the effort it takes to find a sharp knife and a place you are allowed to spit. But $5?

I wheeled my cart past in a fury of "I'm just not going to pay that much for something I used to get two for a quarter."

Once upon a time, I ate whole watermelons in a single sitting.

Big ones, too. Nobody thought anything about digging out the center part and using the rest for slush bombs and seed bullets. When our kids were little, mothers in our neighborhood used to buy half a dozen or so, paint them white and hide them in our yards for an after-supper game with its own built-in prize.

Today, those Dinosaur Egg Hunts would cost $30. Who can afford that on a regular basis?

Besides, even after thumping and smelling and measuring the stripes, you can't really tell until you get in there if you're buying a crispy hunk of heaven or 15 pounds of slimy mush.

Times being what they are now, one just can't make a $5 gamble on something as frivolous as a watermelon. So, I loaded up on Granny Smiths, low-fat yogurt and a bag of lemons.

Watermelon is one of the last summer favorites left on my list.

I gave up coconut Popsicles because of cholesterol, buttered corn because of flabby hips, ditto home-churned peach ice cream and rich milk shakes, Dagwood backyard hamburgers because of blood pressure, Bazooka bubble gum because I'm too old to walk around with sticky lips and gum in my hair, Orange Crush in the dark brown bottles because they quit making them, and fireball jawbreakers because of red dye and a deep cavity in my back molar.

Now I'm being priced out of watermelons. Five dollars today, $10 tomorrow. We might as well cut out summer.

Watermelon is something human beings should have a right to regardless of age, national origin or grocery budget. Even the ancient Egyptians thought so highly of it they immortalized it in pictures on the sides of their tombs.

Not everybody likes it cut in circles, eaten with a spoon and lightly salted, but that's OK. To each his own.

Russians make beer out of watermelon. During the Civil War, the Confederate Army boiled it down as a source of sugar and molasses. According to the National Watermelon Promotion Board in Orlando, Fla., American colonists drank the juice, toasted the seeds and "ate the flesh with relish."

With relish?

I had a cousin who ate watermelon sandwiches on raisin bread, but the closest thing he got to relish was mayonnaise and a pickle. We made him go into the other room to eat.

In 1960, we Americans ate nearly 17 pounds of watermelon per person. That figure is way, way down now. The national average today is about half a watermelon per person.

In my thinking, two things have led to the decline in watermelon consumption.

(No, watermelon doesn't give you consumption, but just you wait. They'll think of something.)

First off, of course, is the rise in cost. But, still, for $5, providing everyone agrees to smaller-than-reasonable portions, you can get at least five slices, or a dollar a serving. That's about what it costs to stir up a gallon of lemonade. Less than a glob of frozen yogurt on a waffle cone. Less than a couple of plastic tomatoes and a heck of a lot more fun than a bag of summer squash.

The real reason watermelon is not as popular as it used to be is because some nitwit biologist has gone public with the fact that it is not a fruit at all. It's a vegetable.

Since then, they just haven't tasted the same.

~ ~ ~ ~ ~

Andy Taylor: "Ready for bed?"
Opie Taylor: "Yes, Pa."
Andy: "Brush your teeth?"
Opie: "Just feel how wet the toothbrush is."
Andy: "I want to tell you a little story. Once, a long time ago, there was this little fella and he never brushed his teeth. Now, you may not believe this, but all he'd do is wet his toothbrush. To him, it was a right funny joke. Every time he thought about it, he'd smile. And then, one day, he quit smilin'. Never smiled again the rest of his days."
Opie: "Why didn't he smile anymore?"
Andy: "He's too embarrassed. He didn't have any teeth."
Opie: "Oh."
Andy: "Where you going?"
Opie: "Guess I'll go brush my teeth again."

Such warmth and wisdom from Mayberry's single-father sheriff explains why there are 12,000-plus members of "The Andy Griffith Show" Rerun Watcher's Club.

DON'T TOY WITH ME

Toy stores make me feel old. What I see is so unlike what I played with and what my children played with, I become hostile and preachy.

Toys started getting complicated with Barbie.

When Barbie was introduced at the 1959 New York Toy Fair, she was a new kind of doll for the American toy chest. In fact, toy buyers thought she was too "chesty," too sexually developed for America's little girls.

That first Barbie cost $3. Today, an original Barbie in mint condition is worth $1,800.

Little girls everywhere were shocked in 1987, when world headlines reported: BARBIE CONVICTED AND JAILED FOR LIFE . . . CRIMES WERE AGAINST HUMANITY. What a relief, when parents explained it was Klaus Barbie they were talking about, not their Barbie.

But nobody seems to mind the subtle crimes and misdemeanors against childhood that Barbie does commit. Perhaps even promotes.

California child psychologist Dr. James Dobson calls Barbie a "role model for anorexia." When a Desert Storm Barbie enlisted as an Air Force pilot, peace organizations all over said, "Now, really!"

Women's groups have a range of complaints, not the least of which is Barbie's unrealistic figure. A woman with those proportions would have to shop for a bra in the circus department, then go down to infant wear to fit her waist.

Not to mention the fact that Barbie and Ken aren't married, even though she's been outfitted with wedding dresses and baby buggies; even though they travel together and move in and out of condos, dream houses and split levels.

Yet Barbie does keep up with the times.

Rollerblade Barbie never falls on her tiny bohunkus when skating into Rollerblade Ken's heart . . . but if she does, she comes with her own fanny pack, which is about the size of one of her mittens.

If you know of any real person whose fanny pack can be the size of her mitten, let me know. I'd like to go on that diet.

For my money, which they will get none of, the real shockers in the toy department are the dolls that make your daughter "pregnant" (does that get your attention or what?), the newest attempt at a child's garden of vulgarity.

Decide for yourself if I'm out of touch here.

Mattel's My Bundle Baby is a pregnancy simulator which enables a little girl — little boys, too, I suppose — to feel the heartbeat, the "kicking" and the excitement of discovering at birth whether it is a boy or a girl.

A company spokeswoman tells us that "Bundle Baby adds another dimension to motherhood."

I'll say.

I've been a mother for 25 years and this is so far out of my dimension, it's way up there in the Twilight Zone.

Kenner's contribution to toy insanity are its Savage Mondo Blitzer action figures. They look like the mutant of a ninja and a hairless King Kong. On skateboards.

Ugly can be cute, but Kenner didn't even get close with the Savage Mondo Blitzers. According to Marianne Szymanski, a toy consultant, if toys are ugly and gross, 6-year-old boys will like them. Kenner went way past "ugly" and "gross." They decided to get downright nauseating. These things have names like Eye Pus, Snot Shot, Puke Shooter, Loaded Diapers and Blood Hockey.

Kenner officials were right pitiful when the snot-snot hit the fan-fan. Thinking parents — even parents with brains slightly larger than a lima bean — started calling the company in protest. Yet Kenner says they got "virtually no complaints" from testing markets before the toys went nationwide.

As the kids say, gimmeee uh break.

Speaking of breaks, the 1992 Toy Fair in New York City featured a whole slew of what-is-this-world-coming-to toys: something called Crash Dummies whereby little kids can set up car accidents and see the bodies fly apart; garbage bags that when dropped in water grow into good-guy and bad-guy creatures; dolls that tan and tee tee in different colors, and trucks that turn into barking dogs.

Toys "R" getting scary.

~ ~ ~ ~ ~

According to Mattel, here — in chronological order — are the careers Barbie has had since 1959:

Fashion model, ballerina, stewardess, candy striper, teacher, fashion editor, flight attendant, medical doctor, Olympic athlete, aerobics instructor, TV news reporter, fashion designer, corporate executive, perfume designer, animal rights volunteer.

DANCE REHEARSAL

Dance is the only art that has no existence outside the human body. The dancer is both paintbrush and canvas, clay and potter, pen and poem.

It can be erotic, hypnotic, secular, sacrificial, rhythmic, rhapsodic, ridiculous. It is a language we learn before birth, as we kick and stretch and squirm, using our bodies to express joy, pain, fear, surprise.

Whether under the moon at Stonehenge, on the streets of New Orleans or in the great theaters of the world, dance is the language of the soul, in all its phases, moods and destinies.

Dance is a verb, a noun, an adjective. And a way of life . . .

"Up . . . lift . . . ankle above the ear . . . keep those hip bones even . . . second, fifth, second, fourth . . . don't just let your feet hang, put energy in them . . . *pas de bourree* . . . hold . . . ”

Neon lights hum a steady base to the one-note rendition of “The Breeze and I” coming from the tape deck in the corner of the studio. Amy Moore Morton, rehearsal mistress for the Appalachian Ballet Company, is taking the dancers through the bar exercises and warm-ups, a nightly ritual for the company's upcoming production of “The Nutcracker.”

What are these dancers thinking? What makes them give up so much? What drives them to starve themselves, to train and practice long hours? To live for their art?

When they try to explain, words don't come easy:

“We take something from very deep inside and try to give it away,” says 17-year-old Amber Gibbons. “I don't know exactly what that ‘something’ is, but it is in every dancer. Sometimes I think of myself as a muse, and it helps me concentrate.”

“I dance with goose bumps all over,” says Morton, 30, cooling down after a breathless series of exercises in preparation for her role as the Sugar Plum Fairy. “There's nothing like it in the world.”

In the waiting room, Sharon Kerr watches her 14-year-old daughter Erika, as Mozart and DeBussy prod Erika through her bar stretches and stances, then turn her loose in a series of floor exercises. In all likelihood, this is Erika's last year as Carla, the child in “Nutcracker” — every up-and-coming dancer's dream role. She has danced the role two previous seasons, but the highlight of her career came this summer when she danced in Act I of “Swan Lake” with the Royal Ballet.

At 25, Michelle Pratt is one of the eight principals with the Appalachian Ballet Company. She works as a bartender, but “dancing is my life.”

“Yes, I worry about getting old. I cried when I turned 25. I can only dance as long as my body allows . . . But if you work every day and love what you are doing — and don't have any injuries —well, I could probably dance into my 40s.”

The warm-up and floor exercises are over. Sweatshirts are tied around their waists. A line forms at the water fountain. Two share a box of Band-Aids. No one is eating a candy bar.

The director claps her hands. The Tchaikovsky tape clicks into place.

There's a last minute tying of shoes and a few quick stretches. The room grows quiet as the director begins the rehearsal by telling them something they all know. By heart.

"Every move, every breath, every hand . . . it's all important. It doesn't take 100 percent . . . it takes 150 percent."

It takes your soul.